ST. ELIZABETHS IN
WASHINGTON, D.C.

ST. ELIZABETHS IN WASHINGTON, D.C.

Architecture of an Asylum

SARAH A. LEAVITT

THE
History
PRESS

Published by The History Press
Charleston, SC
www.historypress.com

Front cover: The Center Building. *Photograph, 1900, National Archives and Records Administration (418-G-7). Back cover*: The Center Building. *Rendering, 2016, U.S. General Services Administration.*

First published 2019

Manufactured in the United States

ISBN 9781467141727

Library of Congress Control Number: 2019932632

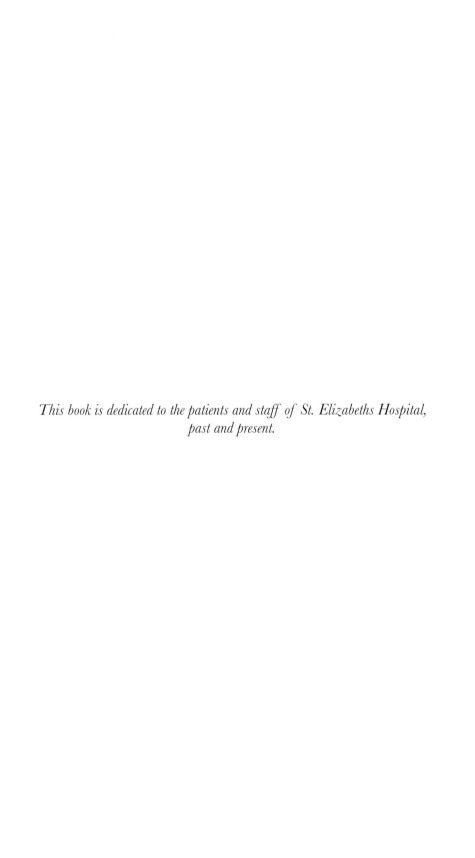

This book is dedicated to the patients and staff of St. Elizabeths Hospital, past and present.

CONTENTS

Preface 9

Introduction 13

PART I: INVENTING THE ASYLUM

Mental Illness 19

The Asylum 22

Dorothea Dix 26

The Kirkbride Plan 28

PART II: THE GOVERNMENT HOSPITAL FOR THE INSANE

The Hospital 35

What's in a Name? 39

The Center Building 41

Gates, Fences, Walls and Roads 49

Landscape 53

Military Connections 56

Cemeteries 59

PART III: A CENTURY OF EXPANSION

Growth 61

The Cottage Plan 62

Howard Hall 67

Godding's Expansion 70

The Richardson Group 73

Mid-Twentieth-Century Expansion 79

CONTENTS

Part IV: Life at St. Elizabeths
Racial Segregation   83
Self-Sufficiency and Farming   87
Hospital Leadership and Staff   94
Recreation   100
Medical Care and Treatment   107
Research   116

Part V: The End of an Era
Deinstitutionalization   123
Kirkbrides Across America   125
D.C. Takes Over   129
St. Elizabeths East   132
The West Campus   139

Epilogue   145
Notes   149
Bibliography   155
About the Author   157

PREFACE

Much of the material in this book was first presented in an exhibition at the National Building Museum in 2017. "Architecture of an Asylum: St. Elizabeths, 1852–2017," on view from March 2017 until January 2018, was curated by Sarah A. Leavitt with Caitlin Bristol, along with other museum staff, interns and the installation team.

Special thanks to many museums and archives for their help, including the St. Elizabeths Hospital Museum, the Stetten Museum, the National Library of Medicine, the National Museum of Health and Medicine, the National Archives and Records Administration and the Library of Congress. The research necessary to create the exhibition and this publication would not have been possible without the preservation of precious and ordinary objects that now help future generations tell the stories of St. Elizabeths.

For their continued work in the historic preservation and redevelopment of the St. Elizabeths West Campus, thanks to the U.S. General Services Administration (GSA), the U.S. Department of Homeland Security (DHS) and the historic preservation advocates and agencies who have consulted on the development of the campus. On the East Campus, thank you to the Deputy Mayor's Office of Planning and Economic Development, as well as the partners of St. Elizabeths East.

With its support of the exhibition and this book, GSA fulfills a commitment for documentation of and public education about the history and architecture of St. Elizabeths, a former federal government hospital for the mentally ill in Southeast Washington, D.C. GSA is developing a consolidated headquarters

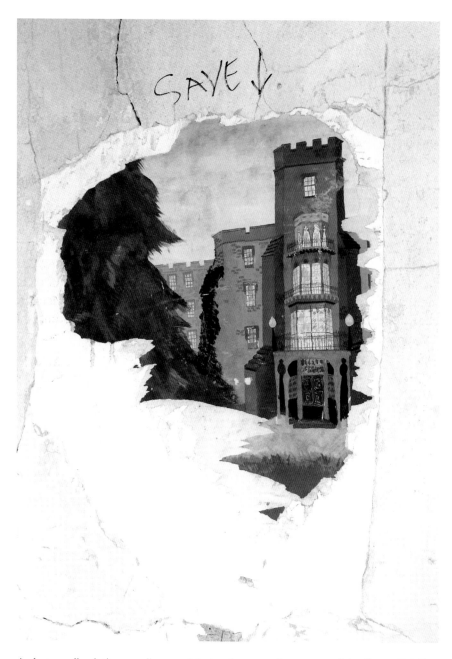

A plaster wall painting was discovered during the renovation process of the Center Building. It was carefully removed, conserved and displayed in the "Architecture of an Asylum" exhibition. *Photograph, 2015, Caitlin Bristol.*

for the DHS on the West Campus of St. Elizabeths, part of a National Historic Landmark District.

The National Historic Preservation Act of 1966 (NHPA) established a program for the preservation of historic properties throughout the United States. Section 106 of the NHPA requires federal agencies to consider the effects of their activities on historic properties. In compliance with NHPA, GSA conducted Section 106 consultation to evaluate the effects of the proposed redevelopment of St. Elizabeths to house the consolidated headquarters of the DHS on the significant historic structures and landscape features that contribute to the National Historic Landmark District.

As part of the Section 106 process, GSA is in ongoing consultation with the District of Columbia State Historic Preservation Office, the Advisory Council on Historic Preservation and other consulting parties on the projects that are implemented as part of the redevelopment of the West Campus of St. Elizabeths. The exhibition and this book were produced in accordance with the 2008 Section 106 Programmatic Agreement governing the redevelopment of the St. Elizabeths Campus and in collaboration with GSA.

INTRODUCTION

America has long struggled with the question of how best to care for the mentally ill. In the mid-nineteenth century, the federal government and many state governments paid to construct and operate specialized buildings to house those with mental illness. They hoped that the architecture and grounds of these facilities, in combination with the care received within, would help lead to a cure. Many of these buildings survive, in part or in whole, and can help tell the story of this era in mental health care.

The Government Hospital for the Insane, later known as St. Elizabeths, opened in Washington, D.C., in 1855 in what is now the Southeast quadrant of the city, near the confluence of the Anacostia and the Potomac Rivers. The hospital grew to become a leader in a national network of public mental health hospitals. Its patient population increased over time, with almost eight thousand people in residence at the height of the hospital's occupancy. Although the Center Building is the most well known of the historic buildings, the hospital was a sprawling campus that once included a working farm and about one hundred structures.

St. Elizabeths is a reminder of a time when the United States led the world in creating and funding an infrastructure to care for the mentally ill. Almost two centuries ago, advocates made heroic efforts to convince state and federal legislators to fund a new movement, known as "moral treatment," to help those with mental illness. Now, the architectural remains of that movement have mostly disappeared. The hospital buildings still on the site in Southeast

Washington are remnants of another era, a time when many believed that the built environment—the buildings and landscapes themselves—could have therapeutic properties. Although it is now understood that buildings, in fact, cannot cure chronic, neurological brain disease, St. Elizabeths' special features indeed offered some measure of hope and improved outcomes for thousands of people. However, funding constraints, overcrowding, misdiagnoses and inadequate treatment complicate the history of the institution.

The grounds and buildings of St. Elizabeths emerged over a period of more than a century, in several stages. Fluctuating ideas about how to best care for the mentally ill guided the architectural choices. The campus evolved from a main institutional building to a series of smaller, Italianate-style cottages; then from a haphazard collection of patient wards and support buildings to grand Neoclassical structures organized around green space; then from one patient building surrounded by abandoned historic structures; to the current plans for two new urban developments for work and living.

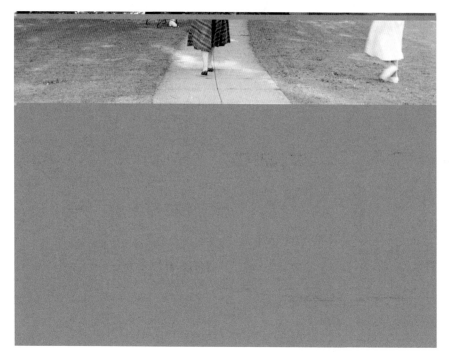

Pathways provide access between buildings for patients and staff. *Photograph, 1955, U.S. National Library of Medicine.*

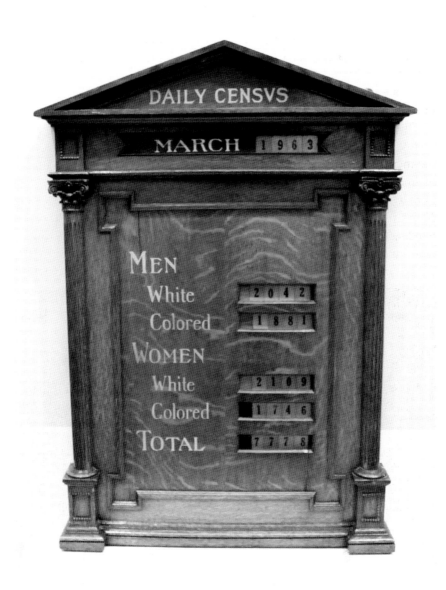

The patient population grew—and grew and grew. This counter tracked the numbers of white and "colored" patients, men and women, at St. Elizabeths. *Census board, circa late nineteenth century, National Museum of Health and Medicine. NBM staff photograph, 2018.*

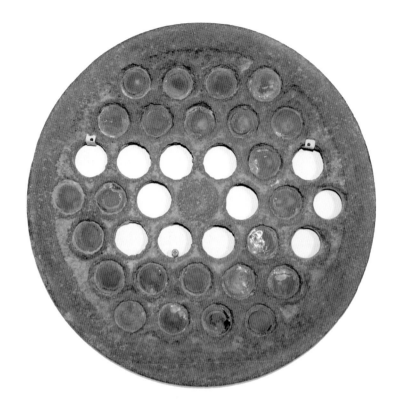

Remains of the old campus, including pieces of infrastructure, continue to help tell the story of the architecture of St. Elizabeths. *Manhole cover, U.S. General Services Administration. NBM staff photograph, 2018.*

St. Elizabeths has been a temporary or permanent home to more than 120,000 patients, from the first patient, Thomas Sessford, who suffered from dementia, to those in care today. Patients' day-to-day lives at St. Elizabeths varied significantly. Some worked on the grounds or in the shops. Many had the opportunity to spend time outside or participate in various activities. However, St. Elizabeths was for its first century a racially segregated campus, and throughout its history, treatment depended on many factors that included race, gender, sexual orientation and severity of diagnosis.

There is still a mental health hospital at St. Elizabeths today that provides care for almost three hundred patients. Although it was a federally run hospital for most of its history, the hospital function of the campus was transferred to the District of Columbia government in 1987. For several decades, D.C.'s hospital operated out of a range of mid-twentieth-century and historic federal buildings, until the modern hospital building opened in 2010. Although the care of mental health patients remains a constant at this site, the current hospital occupies only a small fraction of the historic campus. Today, most of the landscape and buildings at the 350-acre site— half owned by the federal government and half owned by the District of Columbia government—are in the process of real change.

St. Elizabeths tells a story about mental health care, about architecture and landscape architecture and about land use. The history of this hospital and its site is an opportunity to learn more about patients at this particular location and about the treatment of mental illness generally. The United States once invested heavily in institutions to care for a vulnerable population. More than a century and a half later, America struggles with that legacy, both in terms of addressing the future of mental health care and with developing new uses for the buildings that now stand empty across the country. Recent efforts to redevelop St. Elizabeths, designated a National Historic Landmark in 1991, have created new opportunities to access and understand its rich architectural history, as well as its potential to revitalize Ward 8, one of Washington, D.C.'s most underserved areas.

This book explores the history of the hospital's infrastructure. It is one part of a larger conversation about what comes next for Americans with mental illness and the asylums that once served them.

INVENTING THE ASYLUM

MENTAL ILLNESS

A mental illness is a condition that affects a person's thinking, feeling, or mood. Such conditions may affect someone's ability to relate to others and function each day.[1]
—National Alliance on Mental Illness

Researchers have made great strides in understanding the science behind mental illness, although agreement on the care of the mentally ill—both methods and associated costs—is often fraught and complex. For much of human history, in fact, most people considered so-called diseases of the mind to be incurable. The idea to institutionalize the mentally ill in specially designed asylums, sited away from the general population, with the intent to cure them through a specific type of architecture and landscape, was a uniquely mid-nineteenth-century concept. In this period, it was generally understood that mental illness was caused by troubled home life and moral failings and exacerbated by the stressors of modern civilization and industrialization. Many believed that these symptoms could be resolved by removing the patients from their day-to-day lives and relocating them to a calm, bucolic, rural setting with beautiful views, with opportunity for honest hard work and with empathetic treatment.

In the 1850s, when St. Elizabeths opened, mental illness was often characterized in four ways: mania, or "high form," with excitement and

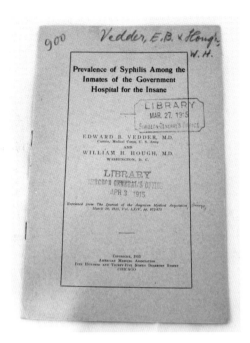

Before the widespread use of penicillin for the treatment of syphilis, many patient admissions were the result of the late stage of the disease. *From Prevalence of Syphilis Among Inmates of the Government Hospital for the Insane, Edward B. Vedder and William H. Hough American Medical Association, 1915, U.S. National Library of Medicine. NBM staff photograph, 2018.*

delusions; melancholia, or "low form," with lethargy and depression; dementia, known as "mental stupor," often caused by brain damage; and monomania, or partial insanity, which could manifest as delusion about one particular subject.

Those sent to public and private mental health hospitals throughout the twentieth century also included "intemperates" (alcoholics), people with untreated epilepsy, elderly people with dementia, those with late-stage syphilis, drug addicts and forensic patients who escaped jail "by reason of insanity" and were remanded to care by the courts. Mental health hospitals also provided respite to many returning from America's wars and suffering from what was once called "shell shock," now known as Post-Traumatic Stress Disorder.

Many hospitals, including St. Elizabeths, admitted gay and lesbian patients for what they called "sexual depravity," as well as heterosexual patients for so-called sexual deviance, which could include promiscuity or sex with unsanctioned partners. Homosexual patients experienced treatments intended to "cure" and treat certain sexual behaviors, especially during the 1940s and 1950s, when the psychiatric profession grew particularly concerned about—and hostile toward—homosexuality. These types of prejudices influenced treatment at St. Elizabeths and

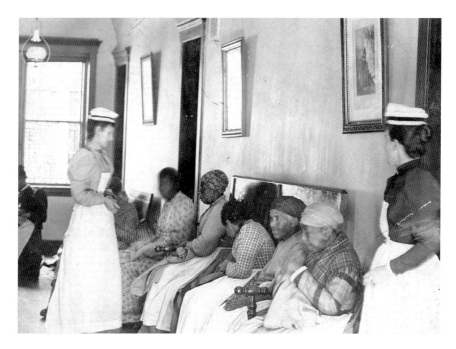

The hospital exclusively employed white attendants and nurses until 1937, and doctors until 1954. *Photograph, 1898, National Archives and Records Administration (418-P-6A-3-1).*

shaped popular understanding of homosexuality as a mental illness for decades to come.

A wide variety of symptoms and diagnoses taxed the resources of many mental health hospitals, where doctors, nurses and attendants worked with patients admitted under a broad—and ever changing—definition of mental illness. Patients could be self-committed, triaged first through a general hospital or arrive through a lunacy proceeding (a jury trial in court). These laws continued to change, with increased emphasis on patient agency, making it increasingly difficult for families and courts to admit a person to a mental health hospital against his or her will.

More research helped practitioners understand the changes in brain function caused by particular disease or trauma. The field of neuropathology, furthered in many ways by work done at St. Elizabeths, reached new conclusions about causes of mental problems. Research gradually led to complex medical knowledge of brain chemistry and the realization that, although many mental illnesses could not be cured, some symptoms could be alleviated.

Today, most mental health researchers agree that mental illness is caused by a combination of factors including genetics and a chemical imbalance in the brain. Issues can arise as the result of abuse, stress and traumatic brain injury. Treatment, then, has progressed considerably over time, based on societal understanding of disease, in-depth research, earlier diagnosis and the availability of resources. While we may have a more modern, scientific understanding of mental illness as caused by brain chemistry, the fundamental ideals of early mental health reformers (fresh air, honest work, empathy on the part of caregivers) are beneficial and still relevant today.

THE ASYLUM

The removal of the insane from home and former associations, with respectful and kind treatment under all circumstances, and in most cases manual labor, [and] *attendance on religious worship on Sunday…are now generally considered as essential in the Moral Treatment of the Insane.*[2]
—Amariah Brigham, March 1847

Mental illness is a medical condition; the asylum is an architectural solution. Those suffering from mental disorders have often been relegated to a separate place, such as a jail or almshouse, to live out their lives away from home. However, architecture was not itself considered part of the cure in most ancient societies. In much of Europe and the United States, this changed in the nineteenth century. The built environment of mental health care has evolved since that time to include many types of structures, from large, sprawling hospital campuses to small outpatient clinics.

One of the first European institutions to accept mental health patients, Bethlehem Hospital, known as "Bedlam," was established in London in 1673 as a home for "poor, senseless creatures." The hospital attended to the needy, especially the "lunaticke."[3] Although not exclusively a hospital for the mentally ill, Bedlam represents the European origins of the concept of separating psychiatric patients from the rest of society. In most places without access to a proper hospital, almshouses or jails served the function of Bedlam. Almshouses were situated in the towns and cities of the British colonies beginning in the seventeenth century. These public buildings to house the poor served many different constituencies.

By the mid-eighteenth century, many colonial cities had begun to regard mental illness as a condition requiring separate treatment in purpose-built hospitals. Specialized facilities opened in a few colonies. One of the British colonies' first mental health hospitals, the Public Hospital for Persons of Insane and Disordered Minds (Eastern Lunatic Asylum), was established by the royal governor of colonial Virginia, Francis Fauquier, in 1773 in Williamsburg. "I should also recommend to your Consideration and Humanity," Fauquier wrote, "a poor unhappy set of People who are deprived of their Senses and wander about the Country, terrifying the Rest of their Fellow Creatures." He recommended "a legal Confinement, and proper Provision…for these miserable Objects, who cannot help themselves."[4] At first, most of these early institutions accepted only white and sometimes free black patients. While institutionalized in these hospitals, patients often met with abusive, brutal or neglectful treatment. Many caretakers resorted to using chains to subdue patients, who rarely recovered from their illnesses.

At the beginning of the nineteenth century, new ideas about healthcare emerged in Europe and around the world, coalescing in a movement known as "moral treatment," with a new type of building at its center. The idea to institutionalize those suffering from mental illness in specialized buildings provided a model for early American asylums. Institutions for orphaned children, tubercular patients, the blind, the elderly, orphans and the disabled were opened to care for those who acted, looked or moved differently from the general population. It was a time when people believed in the power of the asylum to help those in need—but also that removing these people (sometimes against their will) from society was best for them and for the wider community. The asylum was imagined as part of a larger project to impose discipline and order on a rapidly changing and disorderly world. Architects were instrumental in this movement. Soon, institutions across the country connected specific beliefs about mental health care and scientific ideas about the mind with the buildings and landscapes in which healing would take place.

Among the first to establish hospitals specifically for mental illness were Philippe Pinel, at his Bicêtre hospital in Paris, France, and William Tuke at the Retreat in York, England. Both hospitals emphasized recreation and light work in a small, quiet, agrarian setting. The landscape itself was considered to be curative, hewing to the belief that an agrarian lifestyle was healthier than an urban, industrial setting. In America, New Enlightenment intellectuals joined with social reformers to encourage this type of therapeutic regimen. They recommended a new kind of hospital,

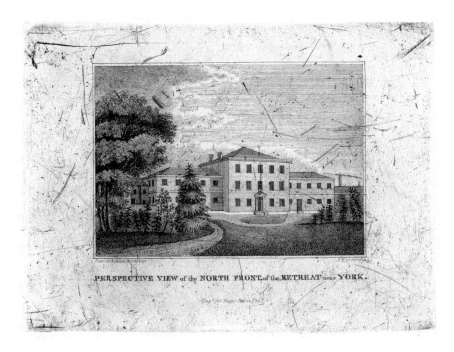

Perspective view of the north front of the Retreat near York. *Drawing, circa 1800, Quaker and Special Collections, Haverford College, Haverford, Pennsylvania.*

combining specialized architecture, empathy and fresh air to restore patients to good health. Moral treatment found its first American advocate in Benjamin Rush in Pennsylvania and soon spread—with the help of mental health advocate Dorothea Dix—across the country.

A period of rapid urban development and change, the nineteenth century saw a rise in the number of mental health patients in the United States, causing an urgent need for new therapies and motivating the government and private hospitals to respond. A dual system of public and private mental health hospitals unfolded as part of the moral treatment movement. Besides a new type of architecture, the moral treatment regimen also included a mandate for humane care, paternalistic oversight and manual labor. By the 1850s, when St. Elizabeths opened, it joined a network of hospitals in states across the country. This state hospital network still exists to some degree, despite small remaining populations of patients.

The mid-twentieth century represented the height of population growth at American asylums, but the tide soon turned. Following advances in drug therapies, a successful patients' rights movement and increased reluctance

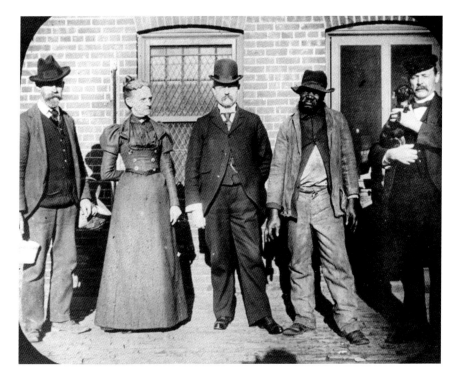

In the late nineteenth century, more than one hundred people worked at St. Elizabeths, including attendants, doctors, housekeepers, cooks, a horticulturist, a kitchen steward, farmers, maids, engineers and carpenters. *Photograph, late nineteenth century, U.S. National Library of Medicine.*

to spend public money on mental health care, deinstitutionalization dismissed many thousands of patients from custodial care. Although patient advocates had imagined that large institutions would be replaced by a network of community mental health centers where people would receive more personal care, this strategy never received enough funding or support to become fully functional.

Today, the National Alliance on Mental Illness estimates that one in five Americans will experience a mental health disorder this year. In lieu of residential care at a mental health hospital, which is significantly rarer now than it was just half a century ago, most of these people will be treated from home with drugs and other therapies; others will stay in hospitals, jails, homeless shelters and prisons, not so unlike the practice of previous centuries. Mental health care advocates contend that between 40 and 60 percent of those currently incarcerated in jails and prisons have had mental health problems.

Unfortunately, many of those with mental illness do not receive the care they need. We still struggle to find answers to what some see as a mental health care crisis. Indeed, although the asylum era became unwieldy, overcrowded and underfunded and was problematic in many ways, looking back on this period and its constructive approaches and idealistic solutions should be part of the national conversation about mental health treatment.

DOROTHEA DIX

We are not sent into this world mainly to enjoy the loveliness therein, nor to sit us down in passive ease; no, we were sent here for action.[5]

—Dorothea Dix

Dorothea Lynde Dix (1802–1887) was an educator and activist who spoke out against the problems in America's mental health care system. In the 1830s and 1840s, Dix traveled across the country to hundreds of jails and prisons, starting in New England. She was disgusted by what she saw as the mistreatment of people suffering from mental illness and made it her life's work to fix what she saw as a breach in the social contract. That is, she believed that the government should help its most vulnerable citizens and was failing in the task. Dix thought, as did many others at the time, that it was specifically the government's role to develop a system of hospitals to provide this care. She worked with state legislatures and with the federal government to implement this plan nationwide and was largely successful.

Dix came to the nation's capital in 1848 with the goal of convincing Congress to use the land grant system to dedicate several million acres for a network of mental health asylums throughout the nation. Land grants had already been used to provide land for public universities and railroads, and she believed that the mechanism could be applied to help the mentally ill. Although her proposition failed—as it had for previous advocates—the government acquiesced in the case of funding a single hospital in Washington and passed legislation in 1852 authorizing the Government Hospital for the Insane.

Although she was the one who proved ultimately successful in securing funding for a federal hospital in Washington, D.C., Dorothea Dix had not been the first to make the argument. In fact, local advocates for a new mental health hospital had been calling for a government-funded facility

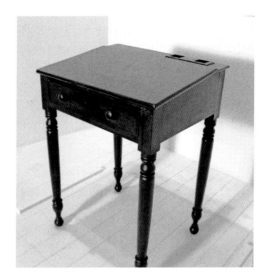

Right: Seated at this desk, Dorothea Dix drafted the legislation to authorize the federal mental health hospital. *Desk, 1850s, Smithsonian Institution, National Museum of American History, Political History Division. NBM staff photograph, 2018.*

Below: As St. Elizabeths reached its 100th birthday in 1955, nurses still admired the pioneering work of founder Dorothea Dix. *Photograph, 1950s, U.S. National Library of Medicine.*

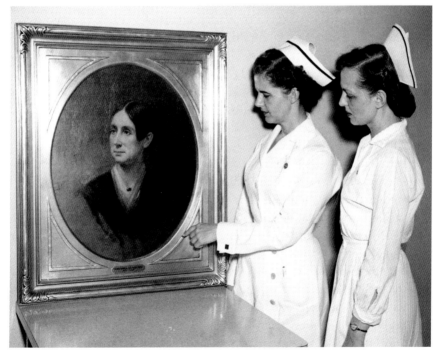

since at least the 1830s. Thomas Miller, the president of the D.C. Board of Health and head of the infirmary at the city jail, was intimately familiar with the problems in housing the mentally ill in the federal city. Miller had tried unsuccessfully to establish a D.C.-based mental health asylum, believing that the number of the mentally ill would continue to grow and that existing facilities in Maryland, where patients had been held, were not prepared to handle the increase. Although D.C. had a smaller population than nearby states, housing mentally ill patients in Baltimore and elsewhere had begun to overtax Maryland's state institutions. Indeed, Dix, having visited Baltimore, testified before Congress about the hospital's overcrowding. Her advocacy, and her friendship with President Millard Fillmore, built on the work of local residents and doctors and finally convinced Congress to act.

Dix remained connected to St. Elizabeths for the rest of her life. In honor of her work, an office was kept for her in the main hospital building. In his 1887 eulogy for the social reformer, St. Elizabeths' first superintendent, Charles Nichols, called Dorothea Dix "the most useful and distinguished woman America has yet produced."[6] Her reputation as a founder of St. Elizabeths endured into the second century of the hospital, and indeed her name graces buildings at hospitals nationwide. Dix is best known as a tireless, and successful, mental health care reformer. As part of her long and varied career, her work in this field stands as a testament to her empathy and perseverance.

THE KIRKBRIDE PLAN

The proper custody and treatment of the insane are now recognized as among the duties which every State owes its citizens.[7]
—Thomas Story Kirkbride, 1854

The Kirkbride Plan was a detailed set of guidelines for the location, arrangement and design of state-sponsored mental health hospitals. Thomas Story Kirkbride (1809–1883), for whom the plan is named, had a major influence on the design of mental health hospitals nationwide, including St. Elizabeths. Kirkbride had extensive experience treating mentally ill patients, having served for several decades as superintendent of the Philadelphia Hospital for the Insane and as founding member of the central professional organization for the field, the Association of Medical Superintendents of American Institutions for the Insane. He had specific ideas about how the built environment could influence medical care. His book, *On the Construction, Organization, and General Arrangements for Hospitals for the Insane* (1854), influenced a generation of architects, planners and hospital superintendents.

In it, Kirkbride outlined theories that he had been honing for more than a decade about the architecture of mental health hospitals, adapting and compiling his ideas from professionals in the field across the country. Kirkbride believed foremost in the temporary separation of the "unsound" from the rest of the general population and in the government's responsibility to provide and pay for those accommodations. He projected that asylums would save the state money in the long run, as this type of incarceration would enable people to recover and later become productive citizens.

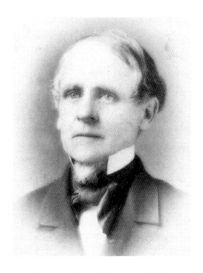

Dr. Thomas Story Kirkbride (1809– 1883) had a major influence on the design of mental health hospitals. *Photograph, circa 1870s, Pennsylvania Hospital Historic Image Collection.*

Central to Kirkbride's philosophy was a specific combination of building and landscape, which dictated the location of each hospital in a rural setting, usually on the outskirts of a city. Kirkbride Plan buildings were designed—by many different architects, on many different types of sites—to be dramatic and beautiful. In the 1830s and 1840s, when Kirkbride wrote his treatise, many Americans lived in rural areas and had never seen a multilevel institutional building. Even in cities, buildings tended to be relatively small and no more than three stories in height. Though large and imposing, Kirkbride structures were intended specifically to look more inviting than a prison, almost resembling outsized country estates. The plan set the ideal capacity of a mental health hospital at 250 patients, so that each occupant could be visited daily by the medical director. Rooms were laid out in stepped-back wings to allow natural light and ventilation as well as unobstructed views. Telltale floor plans with setback wards in a shallow "V" shape, like a bird in flight, characterize a Kirkbride hospital. To impose order on the life of the hospital, patients would be assigned to specific wards based on their race, class and symptoms. The superintendent—as the father figure in a simulated Victorian family setting—would live in the central core building, with women on one side and men on the other. The most severely disturbed patients lived on the wards farthest from the center. Kirkbride believed that hospitals built in this way would best foster a cure.

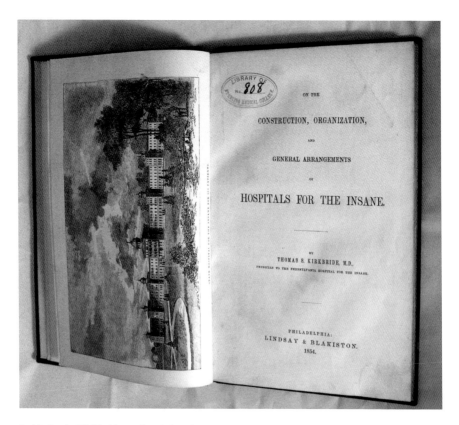

In his book, Kirkbride outlined theories that he had been proposing for more than a decade about the architecture of mental health hospitals. *From* On the Construction, Organization, and General Arrangements of Hospitals for the Insane, Philadelphia, 1854, *Ohio State University, Health Sciences Library, Medical Heritage Center. NBM staff photograph, 2018.*

Kirkbride's ideas spread quickly. Nearly eighty state and local governments opened hospitals for the mentally ill that were designed according to the Kirkbride Plan. Several architects, in fact, became experts at constructing Kirkbride hospitals. Two of the most prolific were Stephen Vaughn Shipman, who designed several asylums in Wisconsin and Iowa, and Samuel Sloan, who worked in New Jersey and Pennsylvania.

Some in the mental health field remained unconvinced by Kirkbride's assurance that asylum design could cure patients. His ideas were new and, in many ways, radical. As early as 1855, John Galt, superintendent at Eastern State Hospital for the mentally ill in Williamsburg, Virginia, published an article criticizing Kirkbride's focus on "studying architecture, in order merely to erect costly and at the same time most unsightly edifices."[8] Galt

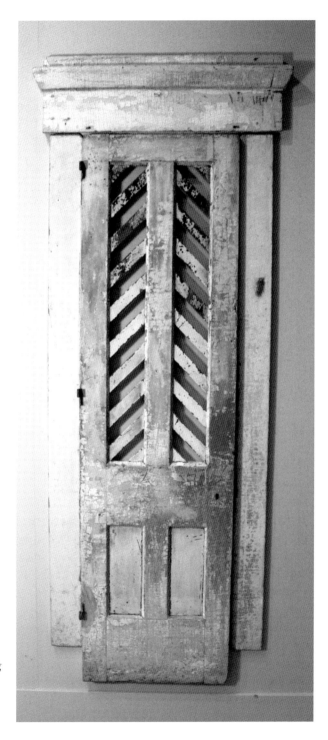

Doors to patient rooms in the Center Building provided some measure of privacy while allowing for ventilation. *Chevron door, U.S. General Services Administration. NBM staff photograph, 2018.*

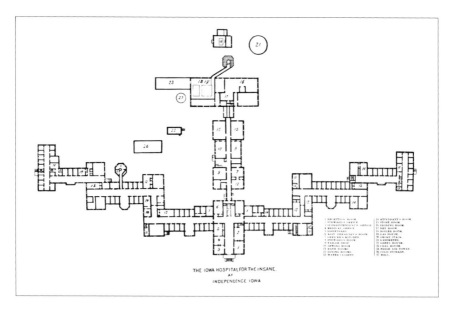

THE IOWA HOSPITAL FOR THE INSANE.
AT
INDEPENDENCE. IOWA

Independence Lunatic Asylum (1873), Independence, Iowa, architect Stephen Vaughn Shipman. *Floor plan, circa 1891, Library of Congress, Historic American Buildings Survey.*

believed in the power of the new talk therapy and even recommended deinstitutionalization—more than a century before America undertook what was then thought to be a revolution in mental health care. For Galt, the best way to treat patients was with drugs, research and other therapeutic activity rather than large custodial institutions. But he was working against the tide in his era.

As it turned out, Kirkbride's philosophy was short-lived in its purest form, although the architectural legacy lived on longer. The numbers of the mental ill continued to grow in American cities despite the new asylums. Even by the 1850s and 1860s, with overcrowding already plaguing brand-new facilities, trust in the Kirkbride Plan was waning. Many state hospitals, especially those in the western states, were founded several decades after the height of the Kirkbride Plan's popularity, and thus their facilities were constructed with different designs. Every state would have a mental health hospital campus by the early twentieth century, but by that time, the complexes were often a compilation of many building types with different architectural styles.

In their attempts to impose order in a rapidly changing world, perhaps the best these hospital administrators could hope for was a measure of control over the burgeoning number of patients with mental illness. In fact, many hospitals followed a similar path: a hopeful opening followed by rapid expansion and deteriorating conditions due to overcrowding and lack of effective treatments.

In the mid- to late twentieth century, new and promising medications allowed for outpatient treatment. A precipitous loss of residential patients, coupled with the loss of public funding, led to the closing of many hospitals. The trajectory of the government-run mental health hospital has for the most part gone from "best hope" to "last resort."

PART II

THE GOVERNMENT HOSPITAL FOR THE INSANE

THE HOSPITAL

There shall be, in the District of Columbia, a Government Hospital for the Insane, and its objects shall be the most humane care and enlightened curative treatment for the insane of the Army and Navy of the United States and of the District of Columbia.[9]

—Civil and Diplomatic Appropriation Act of 1852

In 1852, the U.S. government purchased 185 acres of land that became the bulk of what is now known as the West Campus of St. Elizabeths. Later purchases increased the size of the hospital grounds, most notably the 1869 acquisition of a neighboring farm, now known as the East Campus.

Dorothea Dix had helped to choose the site for the new hospital in the early 1850s. Along with federal government officials, she embarked on a citywide search for a site that would meet Kirkbride's specifications. She wanted to find a spot with a view of the capital city and access to farmable land and water. After scouting the area, they found the St. Elizabeths tract.

By the early 1600s, the area now known as Anacostia included a village called *Nacotchtanke*, probably associated with the local Piscataway tribe. As part of a takeover of land formerly occupied by Native Americans, the British government organized the area into tracts of about one thousand acres each in the 1600s. In 1666, the British granted the St. Elizabeths tract

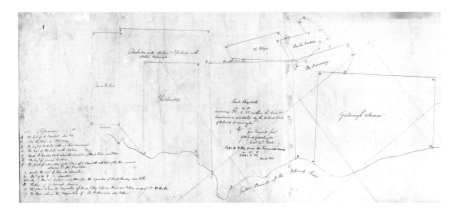

The St. Elizabeths tract was identified as an ideal location for a new institution, providing a rural atmosphere. *Survey map, 1805. Library of Congress, Geography and Map Division.*

to John Charman, who had originally come to the colony as an indentured servant. Over the next centuries, various colonial owners and tenants farmed in the area, which consisted mainly of working tobacco plantations along the Potomac River. The land was annexed into the new federal city in 1790.

St. Elizabeths sits above the confluence of the Anacostia River and the Potomac River, straddling the neighborhoods of Anacostia and Congress Heights in Southeast Washington. The area was outside early development in the capital but provided important services to the city. The nearby Giesboro tract, for example, once a tobacco plantation, became the Giesboro Point Cavalry Depot and supplied Union troops with horses during the Civil War.

Local landowner and lumber titan Thomas Blagden and his wife, Emily Silliman Blagden, acquired the St. Elizabeths parcel in the 1840s. Dix and her government allies, however, approached the couple a decade later with their dreams of building a hospital at the site. To convince the Blagdens to sell, Dix herself spent some time with them, probably walking the land and gazing at the view of the city across the river. Her passion for the St. Elizabeths tract as the perfect site for a mental health hospital was clearly convincing. "Since seeing you today," wrote Thomas Blagden to Dix in 1852, "I have had no other opinion (and Mrs. B also) than that I must not stand between you and the beloved farm."[10] The Blagdens, the last private owners of the site, sold the land to the federal government for $25,000. The Government Hospital for the Insane, designed according to the then-popular Kirkbride Plan for mental health hospitals, first opened on the former Blagden Farm in 1855.

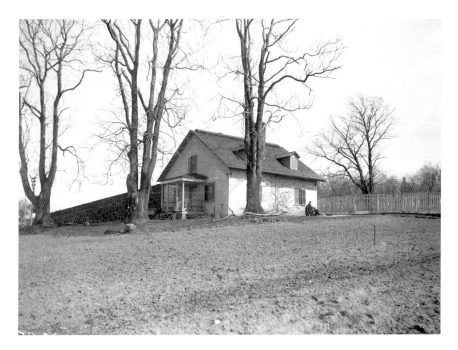

The pleasantly sited St. Elizabeths tract has a long history as a farm and has been owned by several prominent city leaders. The rural acreage continued to be used by the hospital for patient work-therapy, as well as the self-sufficiency of the institution. *Photograph, 1897, National Archives and Records Administration (418-G-118).*

Locating the hospital in an ideal setting within the capital city had been a priority for Dix and other activists. Advocates for the mentally ill believed that asylum grounds should provide a pleasant view, fresh air and plentiful space for farming and outdoor recreation. A distant vista of the growing city—which by then included the yet-unfinished U.S. Capitol building as well as the bustling Navy Yard—maintained separation between the hospital and the stresses of urban life. In the hospital's annual report of 1880, Superintendent William Godding praised the choice of land for incorporating such a magnificent view of Washington, D.C. He noted that for the patients and staff, "there is less of the feeling of isolation when one looks upon the moving panorama of boats upon the river, and there is society in the evening lights of the city beyond; it is the calm presence of the world outside without its distracting roar."[11] Although Washington has changed significantly over the subsequent decades, the expansive views from campus retain therapeutic value.

The hospital was founded under the auspices of the U.S. Department of the Interior, at that time a relatively new federal agency with responsibility

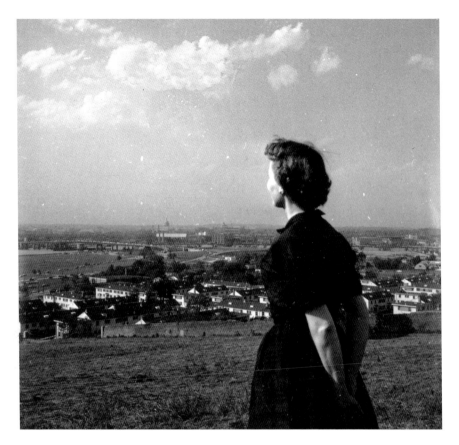

The campus of St. Elizabeths provided a spectacular view of downtown Washington, D.C., including the U.S. Capitol, for the benefit of patients and staff. *Photograph, 1955, U.S. National Library of Medicine.*

for most internal affairs. Interior regulated the federal city's jails and water system, as well as a diverse portfolio of other interests. St. Elizabeths remained under Interior's jurisdiction for almost a century but was transferred to the Public Health Service in 1940 and, from there, to the U.S. Department of Health, Education and Welfare in 1953. Over the next decades, as the city tried to wrest municipal control from the federal government, the hospital passed under the jurisdiction of the National Institute of Mental Health and then to the reformulated U.S. Health and Human Services Department in 1980 before being transferred from the federal government to the District of Columbia's behavioral health department in 1987. Today, there is still a mental health hospital at the site, as there has been since 1855, operated on the East Campus by the government of the District of Columbia.

WHAT'S IN A NAME?

The official stationery of the hospital goes…into thousands of homes, and contains printed thereon reference to the one disease in the whole category of human ailments about which people are most sensitive. It is unnecessary that this should be so, and it could easily be remedied.[12]

—Superintendent William White, 1904

The colonial-era tract on which the hospital was built was known as St. Elizabeths—with no apostrophe. In a coincidental connection to the land's later service to the mentally ill, the area was named in the 1660s after Elizabeth of Hungary, a thirteenth-century Roman Catholic saint who was canonized for her devotion to the poor and the sick. The land changed hands many times, but the original name—inconsistently spelled—stayed connected to the site. Over the course of two centuries, the land passed between owners as tenant farmers, indentured servants and enslaved people raised tobacco and harvested apples on the farm. A survey map from 1805 showed that the site had retained its seventeenth-century name despite changing ownership, as the parcel was marked "St. Elizabeth."

Once the government bought the land, the St. Elizabeths moniker was dropped, at least temporarily. The hospital was officially named the Government Hospital for the Insane, in keeping with conventions to use the word *insane* to describe the mentally ill. However, residents and staff called the hospital St. Elizabeths. During the Civil War, the military located the St. Elizabeth Army General Hospital on the grounds, and recuperating soldiers and sailors used that term for the site. Based in part on the soldiers' and sailors' distaste for the word *insane* in the official name, hospital administration tried for decades to have it changed. However, a formal switch required an act of Congress. In 1916, Congress renamed the mental health hospital to match the colloquial usage.

Indeed, name changes surround the history of the site. The main road, part of the colonial-era King's Highway, was known in the late eighteenth century by the names of various locations along its route: Bladensburg, Piscataway and Giesboro. In 1872, the road was officially renamed to honor Charles Nichols, the first superintendent of St. Elizabeths. A century later, with the site surrounded by African American residential neighborhoods and the city eager to reclaim many federal reservations throughout the capital, Nichols Avenue was renamed Martin Luther King Jr. Avenue in honor of the slain civil rights leader.

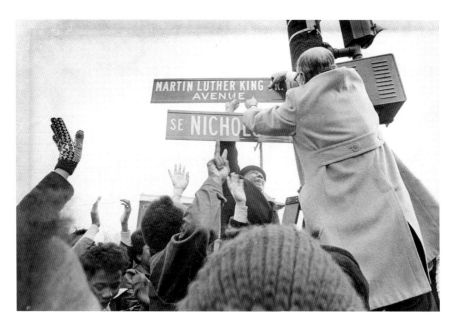

Residents celebrated as Nichols Avenue was renamed Martin Luther King Jr. Avenue in honor of the slain civil rights leader. *From* Evening Star, *"Sign of the Times," January 15, 1971, photograph by Bernie Boston, D.C. Public Library, Star Collection,* © Washington Post.

As the names of the hospital and its main road have changed, so has the language used to describe its inhabitants. The federal facility in Washington, D.C., opened as the Government Hospital for the Insane and is alternately identified on maps as the Government Lunatic Asylum. Today, St. Elizabeths Hospital calls itself a "psychiatric facility for individuals with serious and persistent mental illness." Although words like *insane*, *crazy*, *idiot*, *moron* and *lunatic* were once regularly used, they are now considered disrespectful and inappropriate. Today, phrases like "mental health," "patient with mental illness" and "psychiatric care" are changing over to language that highlights the agency of the person receiving care. Many service groups and mental health advocates use the term *consumer* or the phrase "person with lived experience" to describe a person in care at a residential hospital.

THE CENTER BUILDING

It is the desire of the President that the proposed hospital shall be a model institution, embracing all improvements which science, skill, and experience have introduced into modern establishments.[13]
—Alexander H.H. Stuart, Secretary of the Interior, 1852

The Center Building was St. Elizabeths' first and most impressive edifice and was purposefully designed with aspirations to serve the nation as a model institution. Superintendent Nichols described the building's relatively plain, practical style to Congress as resembling a castle or a villa, but in a "collegiate gothic style…highly effective, in view of its plainness and the cheapness of the materials in which it can be represented."[14] The imposing structure, built in red brick with sandstone detailing in a blend of the then-popular Italianate and Gothic Revival styles, followed the Kirkbride Plan with its large central tower at its core flanked by stepped back wings.

The building incorporated mid-nineteenth-century architectural details such as a full-height projecting bay with Gothic window tracery. Hundreds of tall double-hung sash windows surmounted by label moldings were characteristic of a then-popular residential architectural style. The structure also featured parapets, buttresses and cast-iron railings. A Victorian-era porte-cochère, rebuilt in the 1930s, protected visitors arriving in carriages from the weather while adding distinction to the building's façade. The main structure, built for white patients, sustained many additions over several decades, beginning with the west wing in 1855, through the Willow building in 1895, eventually attaining a length of nine hundred feet.

Thomas Ustick Walter (1804–1887), the federal government's Supervising Architect of the Treasury, was the architect of the Center Building. He is best known for his service as the fourth architect at the U.S. Capitol Building, for which he designed the north and south wings in addition to the distinctive dome. Walter had been appointed architect of the Capitol extension by President Millard Fillmore in 1851, making him well poised for the St. Elizabeths job, since Fillmore had been working with Dorothea Dix on the preparations for the site. Walter had previously worked on large institutional structures, such as Girard College for Orphans in Philadelphia (1832). After his work in Washington, Walter returned to Philadelphia, where he worked with the architect of the city hall in the 1870s and 1880s.

At St. Elizabeths, Walter had several patrons to please. Superintendent Nichols was heavily involved with the design and construction of the Center

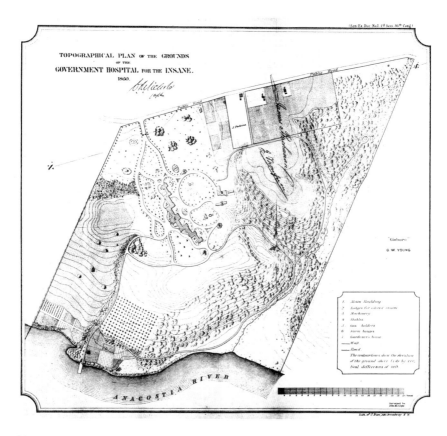

This early site plan shows the placement of the hospital's first buildings surrounded by trees, farmland and a ravine. *From the Annual Report, 1860, Library of Congress, American Architectural Foundation Collection.*

Building. The new superintendent arrived in Washington in 1852—years before there was a hospital built or any patients—with the intent to consult on the construction of the first several structures. He served as, essentially, a general contractor on the job, leaving behind extensive correspondence concerning everything from bags of sand to nails. He sent the architect sketches of his ideas, requesting that the main building "blend architectural beauty with practical convenience and utility."[15] Walter and Nichols worked together to modify Kirkbride's recommended design, adding perpendicular corridors between each ward to isolate patients and reducing the capacity of the farthest wards to limit the admission of severely disturbed patients.

Construction itself took several years. As described by Superintendent Nichols in his 1860 report to Congress, "certain strong patients of the

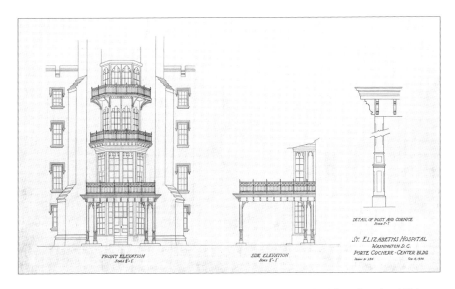

This ornamental porte-cochère welcomed visitors to the Center Building. *Drawing, 1938, Library of Congress, American Architectural Foundation Collection.*

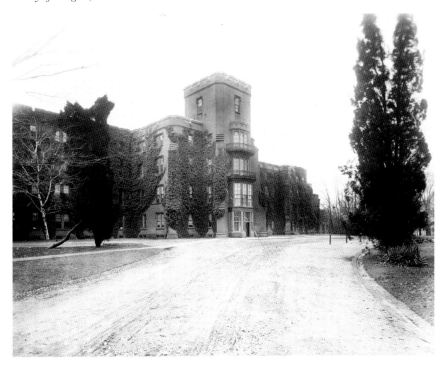

Patient wards took up most of the floors in the Center Building, with the superintendent's office and family quarters occupying rooms on the second and third floors of the center tower. *Photograph, circa 1910, Library of Congress, Prints & Photographs Division.*

laboring class"[16] dug clay from the grounds and formed the bricks for the Center Building complex. The workers had produced more than 9 million bricks by 1860. In part because patients did much of the labor themselves, construction was slow-going. Residents of the Center Building, therefore, lived for many years in an unfinished hospital. In a report to the board of directors in 1858, Nichols described the construction in progress: "All the walls of the Center have been raised to their full height. The rear exterior walls had reached the foot of the 3rd story."[17] Laborers harvested wood from trees found at the site, which purportedly inspired the names for the Oak, Ash, Poplar, Cherry and Birch hospital wings. Iron doors, used for fire safety as well as patient containment, separated the wards. Ever interested in reducing costs, Nichols even repurposed old fencing from the Giesboro Cavalry Depot after the Civil War.

As dictated by Kirkbride, the central core of the building housed the superintendent's apartment and administrative offices. The Center Building's layout allowed for separation of patients by diagnosis, a feature fundamental to the Kirkbride Plan. Patients with more severe symptoms who might act out or be unable to modulate their volume lived on the outer wards, while those with milder symptoms occupied rooms closer to the administrative offices and living quarters in the center. The wards, which had separate staircases to allow for safety and privacy, decreased in size toward the ends of the building, with those farthest from the center having no parlors or common rooms. The walk from one end of the building to the other was long and involved several doors and corridors, helping to ensure the boundaries between patients held fast.

Decoration in patient rooms varied widely in the nineteenth century depending on the severity and type of illness, as well as a patient's wealth. According to Nichols's recommendations, furniture on the wards was designed to be durable in order to be "most safe in the hands of a household of insane persons."[18]

Overcrowding was a constant problem in the Center Building. As early as the 1870s, patients were doubling and tripling up in single rooms. Although the structure was built with the idea of an even male/female split, St. Elizabeths' status as the mental health hospital for the army and the navy meant that more than half of its patients were veterans—all of whom were men—and thus the hospital had an unequal balance of men and women from its earliest decades. This had implications for women, who had less freedom to move around the campus, and for men, who lived in increasingly overcrowded conditions. Nichols tried to push for an all-female building on

Right: Workers dug clay from the grounds and produced more than 9 million bricks by 1860. *Bricks from the Center Building, circa 1850s, U.S. General Services Administration. Photo by Yassine El Mansouri, 2017.*

Below: This brick reveals evidence that a dog interrupted construction of the Center Building. *Brick, circa 1850s, found in kiln excavation, 2015, U.S. General Services Administration. NBM staff photograph, 2018.*

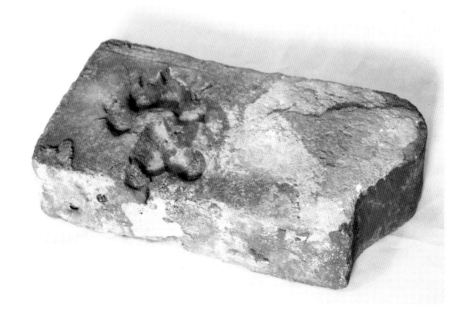

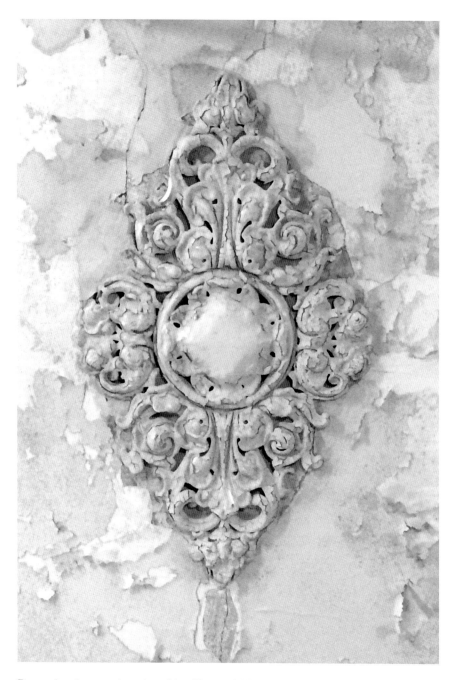

Decorative plasterwork, such as this ceiling medallion in a hallway of the Center Building, was carefully documented and repaired or replicated. *Photograph, 2015, Caitlin Bristol.*

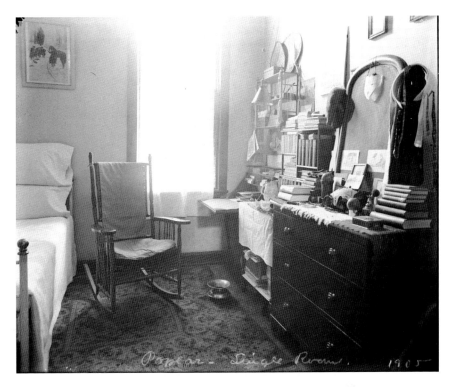

Decoration in the Center Building patient rooms varied widely in the nineteenth century, depending on factors including the severity and type of illness. *Photograph, 1905, National Archives and Records Administration (418-G-223).*

the more secluded East Campus in 1876—in part to give women the chance to walk outside more freely—but the request was denied by Congress. In 1876, 176 men (out of a total male population of 550) slept on mattresses pulled into the wide corridors.

The Center Building was a practical structure that incorporated service functions as well as patient rooms, administrative offices and living quarters. A system of tracks enabled a small narrow-gauge train car system to carry food, laundry and other supplies throughout the building. Later, underground tunnels also connected the Center Building to other buildings on campus.

A modern coal-fired gravity system heated the Center Building by circulating hot water throughout the structure. Kirkbride devoted an entire chapter of his influential book to the best ways to carefully regulate airflow and ventilation in such a large structure. He noted that open-hearth fires were the most pleasant heating mechanism. This innovation replaced often

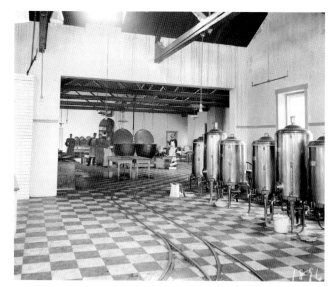

The Center Building was a practical structure that served hundreds of patients. A system of tracks and tunnels ferried food from the kitchen throughout the building. *Photograph, 1896, National Archives and Records Administration (418-G-176).*

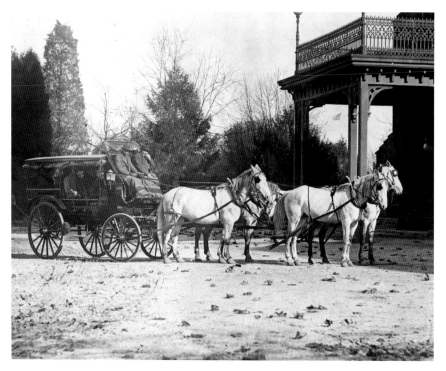

The decorative porte-cochère at the Center Building provided coverage for visitors after a horse and carriage ride. *Photograph, nineteenth century, U.S. National Library of Medicine.*

dangerous and inefficient fireplaces since, according to Kirkbride, "the risks attending them, at times, even in the least excited wards, are so numerous as to render it prudent to dispense with them."[19]

The Center Building, constructed by patients and local workers and designed by one of Washington, D.C.'s most important architects, symbolized the federal government's investment in housing and protecting the mentally ill. However, its promise was soon overshadowed by new ideas in psychiatry about how to best house patients. In 1866, only a decade after the Center Building welcomed its first residents, the political leadership of the mental health field, the Association of Medical Superintendents of American Institutions for the Insane, officially changed the recommendations for the construction of hospitals. Instead of suggesting that patients could be cured in a particular kind of building, the new mandate shifted away from the Kirkbride Plan. Leaders in the field now held a more pragmatic understanding of the custodial role of the mental health hospital campus in the age of chronic disease. The new regulations called for larger populations—600 rather than 250—and smaller buildings for living quarters.

GATES, FENCES, WALLS AND ROADS

All concerned feel that few expenditures give more satisfaction than those for properly enclosing the grounds of a hospital.[20]

—Thomas Kirkbride

St. Elizabeths occupies a wide swath of land on a bluff overlooking the city, with a view of both the Potomac and Anacostia Rivers. However, the land has been walled off from the rest of Washington for more than a century and a half. Although thousands of patients and staff members once lived there—and thousands of people work there today—most of the city's current residents and tourists have never been behind the walls and fences that surround the hospital campus.

Walls and fences serve many historic and contemporary purposes, including keeping patients in, keeping residents out and keeping both safe from one another. The high-level government offices now located on the campus necessitate a secure boundary around the site. Thomas Kirkbride himself believed that the wall or fence should serve more as a visual barrier than a true deterrent to escape and should not replace attendants and other

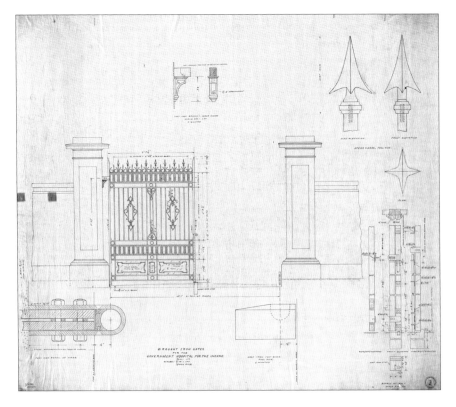

In 1912, after much growth on the hospital campus, a report to the Department of the Interior suggested improvements to the fence surrounding the hospital. *Drawing, 1912, Library of Congress, American Architectural Foundation Collection.*

staff in keeping the patients safe. Indeed, the hospital was to not look like a prison but was also to remain separate from the surrounding community.

Of course, the barrier has always been porous. Over time, some patients had privileges to leave the campus, and neighborhood residents could attend lectures, movies and other performances. Workers and suppliers traveled through the area daily. Although many staff members lived on campus, they entertained guests who entered through the gates. Curious area residents and those looking for a shortcut through the neighborhood found reason to walk through the property. But throughout the hospital's history, a combination of gates, fences and walls made up a physical boundary around the grounds of St. Elizabeths.

Superintendent Nichols began construction of the first wall around the campus in 1859, assuring Congress that the wall kept patients "in perfect freedom from molestation from without, and without the invitation to

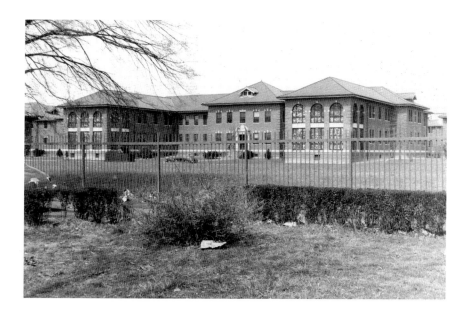

These photographs illustrate the view of the hospital from the perspective of its neighbors in Congress Heights. *Photographs, 1950, John P. Wymer Photograph Collection, Historical Society of Washington, D.C.*

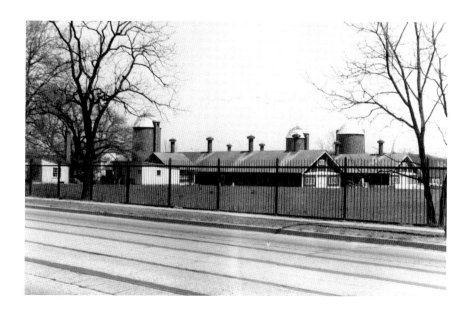

escape."[21] Stone for the wall was quarried from nearby Barry Farm. The wall surrounded the campus on all sides, including a segment that traveled 150 feet into the Potomac River to help deter entrance by boaters and fishermen.

As the area was fairly remote from the center of the city, roads leading to and from campus were limited in the hospital's early years. Superintendent Nichols implored Congress to improve Asylum Road (today's Martin Luther King Jr. Avenue, SE) to provide better, more reliable all-weather access between the hospital and downtown. The meager local population on the east side of the Anacostia River meant that Congress was wary to spend money on infrastructure. Eventually, however, proximity to the Giesboro Cavalry Depot convinced the government to provide a new road. Nichols himself organized the labor, whom he gathered from the area, including the use of so-called contraband, or men who had escaped slavery. The road was later renamed Nichols Avenue in his honor.

By 1912, after much growth on the hospital campus, an administrative report to the Department of the Interior suggested improvements to a fence

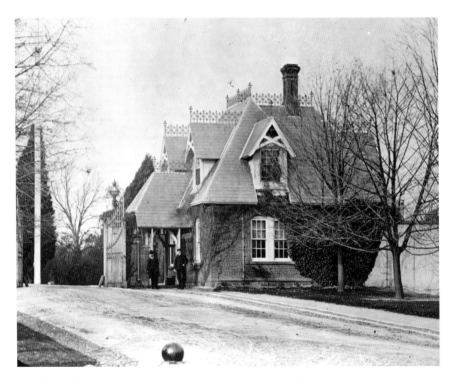

The Queen Anne–style gatehouse to the campus provided welcome to visitors and security for patients. *Photograph, 1874, National Library of Medicine*

that "should surround the hospital grounds" even more securely than the original wall. To discourage trips into town, an old farm building was used by St. Elizabeths as a canteen for those patients who had earned the privilege to walk around with relative freedom. One motivation for opening an on-campus store was to control purchases; local businesses had been selling patients forbidden items such as matches and knives.

Several gatehouses provided security for the hospital as formal visitor entry sites and demonstrate the changing architectural styles on the campus. Gatehouse No. 1, the oldest of these structures, was constructed in the picturesque Queen Anne style. Bronze-colored eagles, long a symbol of American pride and power, guard the hospital gates. Another gatehouse, dating from 1926, is a one-story brick structure with an overhanging roof. A gatehouse built in 1958 is a single-story utilitarian structure with metal windows and corrugated metal siding, contrasting with the earlier campus entrances.

LANDSCAPE

The building should be in a healthful, pleasant, and fertile district of the country; the land chosen should be of good quality and easily tilled; the surrounding scenery should be varied and attractive.[22]

—Thomas Kirkbride, 1854

Landscape design played an important role in the medical treatment goals of St. Elizabeths. The hospital was part of a larger backlash to industrialization that considered a pastoral landscape to be an antidote to the pressures of modern life. An early site plan shows the placement of the hospital's first buildings surrounded by trees, farmland and a ravine. However, despite the belief that the ideal recovery included peaceful nature walks and views, St. Elizabeths was constantly growing and perpetual campus construction produced disruptive sounds and detours.

In the nineteenth century, mental health experts associated illness with the troubles of the modern, urban world. In a report to Congress in 1855, Superintendent Nichols waxed poetic about the bucolic hospital where "changing and ever grateful beauties of trees, shrubs, and flowers, amid walks and parterres" would help separate the "diseased mind from its delusions."[23]

In the 1880s, after the purchase of the East Campus, which was then mostly farmland, Superintendent Godding described an agricultural utopia in which patients could live in farmhouses, work with animals and cultivate the land. However, although some patients did spend time on the farm over the course of the next few decades, this grand vision never fully came to pass. Plans for a patient colony were thwarted by delays in finding a source of potable water, and patients always lived in large residential halls, not farmhouses. However, Godding repeatedly asked Congress for money to buy more land, believing that a hospital should have one acre of land per patient—a figure that became more and more impractical as the decades passed.

The opportunity to spend extended time outside varied among patients, although many did take regular therapeutic walks and do outdoor exercises. Bird baths, water fountains and summer houses, or small gazebos, encouraged some patients to walk outdoors. Water features on campus included a duck pond and a water fountain along the south side of the Center Building. Benches throughout campus provided places for infirm or tired patients to sit down and relax.

A new landscape design after the Civil War improved the drives and walkways. The prevailing belief in the benefits of planned gardens led to the reshaping of the natural grounds into a carefully landscaped setting. Superintendent Nichols oversaw the planting of one thousand trees in the early 1860s and turned twenty-five acres of the site into cultivated lawn. Five hundred shade trees donated by the Parking Commission of Washington, D.C., enhanced the comfort of new paths. Beyond these decorative paths and plantings, rural farmland surrounded the hospital.

Longtime master gardener Alvah Godding, son of the hospital's second superintendent, laid the groundwork for extensive gardens with trees and plants gathered from around the world. The younger Godding grew up on the grounds of the hospital and stayed on to serve the institution as superintendent of the grounds from the 1890s through 1949, well after his father's tenure. While superintendent, William Godding had expanded and improved the greenhouses to provide work for patients, as well as flowers for patient wards. His son, inspired by international travels, planted flowers, trees and bushes for the enjoyment of patients and staff. In front of the Center Building, the hospital planted trees not native to the eastern United States, including Japanese torreya, giant sequoia and Japanese cryptomeria.

In the 1920s, concrete roads, pathways and curbs brought the campus into the modern era, as increasingly vast areas of landscaping gave way

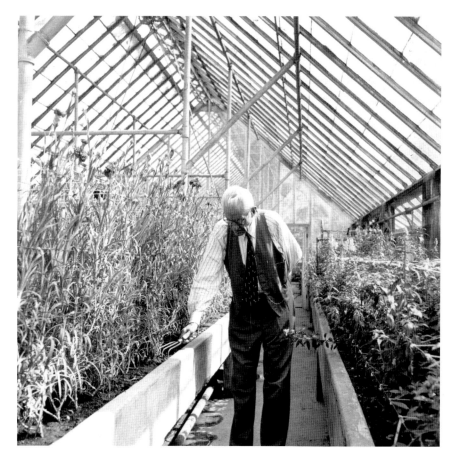

Longtime master gardener Alvah Godding, son of the superintendent, established extensive gardens with trees and plants gathered from around the world. *Photograph, 1955, U.S. National Library of Medicine.*

to pavement in the form of driveways, sidewalks and parking lots. Cars and trucks changed the character of the rural site. As cars became more important to maintaining the grounds, transporting staff and supplies and other logistical uses, the campus built its first garage—a white, modern building with large glass-brick windows. Cars forced other changes to the grounds as well, especially the paving of formerly green areas for roads and parking lots. In the 1950s, the construction of the Anacostia Freeway (now Interstate 295) resulted in a fifteen-acre loss for the hospital grounds. Despite the changes, thickets of trees and sweeping views continued to provide some rural character to the site.

MILITARY CONNECTIONS

St. Elizabeths originally admitted patients from three populations: the U.S. military, through the army and the navy; those living on federal land nationwide such as Indian reservations; and residents of the District of Columbia. The military relationship meant that individuals could be transferred directly from service—or from the branches of the National Home for Disabled Volunteer Soldiers, if care there was not sufficient. Over the century-long association with the military, usually more than half of St. Elizabeths patients at any given time were veterans. Although Superintendent Godding tried in the late nineteenth century to annex additional land for the purpose of separating military patients from civilians, this never came to pass.

Only six years after the hospital opened, the Civil War began to rage nearby. The Union Army established its headquarters in Washington, so the government constructed dozens of military hospitals, army forts and navy bases throughout the city and requisitioned other buildings for medical care. In addition, an average of twenty thousand Union troops were billeted in and around the capital for its protection during the war. By the end of the conflict, the city was fortified with an extensive defense system and a network of hospitals, including St. Elizabeths. The site housed convalescing or recuperating soldiers and sailors both as mental patients and in its temporary role as a general military hospital. During the conflict, St. Elizabeths also became an integral part of Washington, D.C.'s military network as a site for artillery training.

The campus quickly filled with tents for convalescing patients, but this was not the only change to the landscape. The Pen Cote Battery was one of many new or temporary defensive structures, while other buildings were retrofitted for army and navy usage. Almost two thousand sick and wounded soldiers and sailors lived temporarily in the unfinished east wing of the Center Building, in the West Lodge for African American patients and in tents on the grounds. The gardener's cottage became a quarantine hospital for patients with infectious diseases. Well past the years of the war, the cemetery at St. Elizabeths filled with iron crosses and military-issued headstones marking new graves.

The most significant Union casualty to recuperate at St. Elizabeths was General Joseph Hooker, who spent time there recovering from a gunshot wound inflicted at the Battle of Antietam in September 1862. He was personally attended to by Superintendent Nichols in the Center Building.

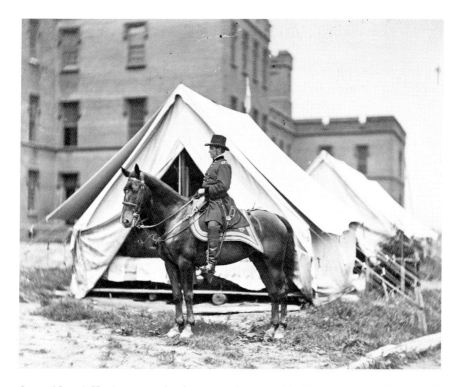

General Joseph Hooker, recovering from a gunshot wound in 1862, was personally attended to by Superintendent Nichols in the Center Building during the Civil War. *Photograph, circa 1860s, Library of Congress, Prints & Photographs Division.*

Hooker recovered and went on to lead Union troops in later battles. President Abraham Lincoln, who spent time visiting his soldiers throughout the city, came to visit General Hooker and presumably other convalescing veterans.

In 1863, in the middle of the war, B.W. Jewett established a St. Elizabeths outpost of his Washington, D.C.–based artificial limb manufacturing shop to serve military amputees. Soldiers and sailors from neighboring hospitals were transferred to St. Elizabeths to be fitted with prostheses and to recover from their wounds and learn how to use their new limbs. The operation was relocated in 1864 due to overcrowding.

The connection between St. Elizabeths and the military continued well after the Civil War. Serving a large in-house population of veterans, St. Elizabeths rose to the forefront of the emerging field of military psychiatry. The Spanish-American War saw an increase in patient admissions from Manila, San Juan and Santiago in the late 1890s. After World War I, thousands of veterans suffering from what was then called "shell shock"

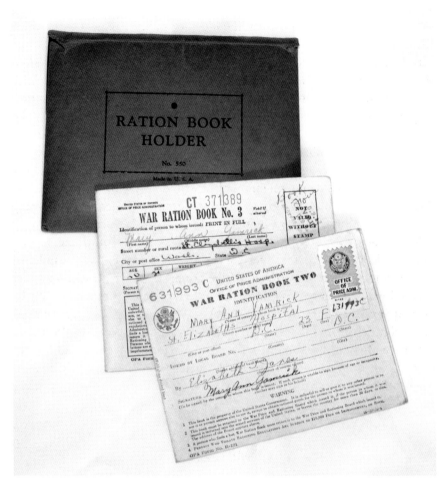

Nurses, caretakers and other staff at St. Elizabeths during World War II had to use ration books for basic supplies just like the world outside the fence. *World War II ration book, 1940s, St. Elizabeths Hospital Museum. NBM staff photograph, 2018.*

came to St. Elizabeths. As a volunteer for the American Red Cross, Eleanor Roosevelt visited the hospital, where she found thousands of convalescing soldiers and sailors who had returned suffering from tremors, confusion, panics and nightmares. The hospital's overcrowded and antiquated conditions horrified Roosevelt. She encountered despondent and neglected veterans and aging facilities, all of which were far from what the hospital's founders had envisioned. After her visit, Roosevelt urged Secretary of the Interior Franklin Lane to launch an investigation into conditions at St. Elizabeths. She also lobbied Congress to increase funding to the hospital.

Her efforts resulted in an increased budget for military patient care, which led to the construction of the so-called semi-permanent structures on the East Campus. These seven temporary patient wards, housing five hundred people each, lasted for decades but were finally demolished in the mid-1940s.

World War II brought thousands of veterans to the hospital with a new diagnosis, Post-Traumatic Stress Syndrome. By this time, however, the nation's system of Veterans Administration hospitals had begun to assume responsibility for military healthcare. Patients were often triaged at St. Elizabeths before being sent to other institutions. The growing availability of alternatives meant that military patients could be admitted to hospitals in their home states, making visiting easier for family members and spreading out the burden of care throughout the country.

The official relationship of St. Elizabeths hospital and the armed forces ended in 1946, after ninety-one years. The severing of the military connection changed the makeup of the patient population. Although the hospital was able to relocate several hundred patients—freeing up much-needed space—its remaining population skewed older and experienced more chronic mental illness. The loss of the military patients also made it harder for hospital administrators to petition Congress for additional funds. The hospital, now increasingly focused on the local population, began its trajectory out of the federal orbit.

CEMETERIES

St. Elizabeths has two cemeteries, both of which include the graves of military veterans and civilians. The West Campus cemetery was in use for about two decades, until 1874, and contains approximately 500 graves, a number that includes 220 Civil War veterans who were patients at the hospital. The grave markers were placed after the war and were moved several times in the following years so that they no longer necessarily correspond to individual grave sites.

The East Campus cemetery opened in 1873 and contains the graves of 2,050 military veterans and more than 3,000 civilians, including 14 patients who had been transferred to St. Elizabeths from the Hiawatha Asylum for Insane Indians. The cemetery grounds on the East Campus also included a cottage, or sexton house, providing rooms for the on-site caretaker.

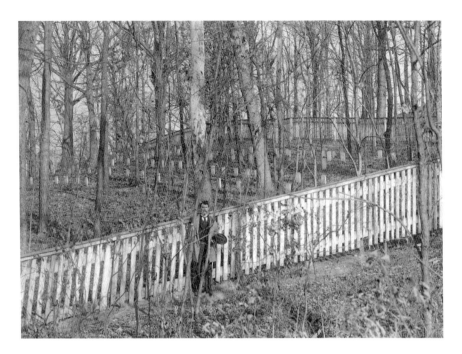

The West Campus cemetery became inactive in 1874 and comprises approximately 500 graves, including 220 Civil War veterans who were patients at the hospital. *Photograph, 1897, National Archives and Records Administration (418-P-544).*

Mental health hospitals across the country are the final home to thousands of so-called friendless patients who lie in unmarked graves. At Oregon State Hospital's Building 60 in Salem, for example, the public can visit the cremated remains of 3,423 unnamed patients. At St. Elizabeths, because it served the entire nation as one of the only federal mental health hospitals, some mental health advocates hope to construct a memorial on the East Campus to patients who rest in unmarked graves, honoring those at public mental health hospitals throughout the country.

PART III

A CENTURY OF EXPANSION

GROWTH

The question for us is no longer whether the hospital for a large or a small number is the best ideal provision for the insane, but how shall we manage to take care of what we now have and of the increasing number who are every year pouring in upon us.[24]

—Superintendent William Godding, 1891

St. Elizabeths grew in ways that were both typical of other hospitals nationwide and unique to its position as a federal facility. The first iteration of the campus was completed in 1855 to house a population of 250 patients and was almost immediately overcrowded. For its entire first century, constant increase in the number of patients, a growing emphasis on science within the mental health field, the types of diseases encountered and congressional funding all propelled the construction of additional buildings at the hospital. Mental health advocates, with dreams of curing patients and sending them home, instead faced an expanding population of the chronically mentally ill.

Indeed, all American mental health hospitals—both private and public, everywhere across the country—experienced rapid, exponential growth throughout the first half of the twentieth century. General population increase, family dislocation caused by migration, hardship during the Great Depression and increased trust in institutional care were all factors. New diagnoses and changes in the definition of mental illness—as well as the rise of certain diseases, including neurosyphilis and alcoholism—led to more and more people needing residential care. The numbers of so-called criminally insane, or forensic patients, increased nationwide as well, as the courts remanded patients to care either while awaiting trial or after a verdict. Patients with chronic illnesses taxed the resources of all hospitals, demanding all the more structures to house them.

St. Elizabeths also had some uniquely specialized populations not necessarily experienced by state hospitals nationwide. The institution took in military patients from all across the country, with a high number of war veterans suffering from "shell shock." Also, as the mental health hospital for the federal government, St. Elizabeths brought in a new population of Native Americans after the Canton Asylum for Insane Indians was shut down by the Department of the Interior in 1933.

The hospital's organizational structure and physical development followed larger nationwide trends in scientific study, farming and civic building design. New architectural approaches became necessary as the hospital expanded in stages. In the late nineteenth century, the Cottage Plan introduced small-scale, specialized buildings and farm structures. At the turn of the twentieth century, an organized development plan brought Neoclassical order to the institutional landscape. An increased focus on scientific research led to a new laboratory, while a decreased emphasis on farming and loss of land led to new patient wards.

THE COTTAGE PLAN

Driven partly by shifting ideology and partly by economic realities, leaders in the mental health field in the late nineteenth century began advocating for a new model of patient care: a homelike setting in a series of buildings rather than one centralized institutional structure. First incorporated on a major scale by the Kankakee State Hospital in Illinois, the Cottage Plan rapidly overtook the Kirkbride Plan as the go-to choice for institutional design nationwide.

By the 1880s, St. Elizabeths' second superintendent, William Godding, had become a national advocate for the new cottages. He and other psychiatric doctors increasingly argued that a more domestic environment best suited the needs of chronic patients, who might live most of their lives on the hospital grounds. Superintendent Godding called this transition to the dormitory-style cottages "the end of the cathedral era" and oversaw the construction of more than a dozen Cottage Plan buildings, built in a residential-scale, Victorian style. This new system was just as short-lived as the Kirkbride model, however. After the turn of the century, the architectural paradigm shifted back in favor of large patient buildings, encompassing some of the features of both the Kirkbride and the Cottage Plans.

Atkins Hall, constructed in 1878, was the first Cottage Plan building at St. Elizabeths. Many of the cottages at St. Elizabeths were built in a similar architectural style in an attempt at visual homogeneity. Yet rather than conform to a quadrangle arrangement or other formal site plan, these detached buildings were haphazardly placed in relation to the Center Building.

Atkins Hall was originally intended for quiet, white, working-class, male patients. The building was named for John DeWitt Clinton Atkins, the congressional representative from Tennessee who helped appropriate

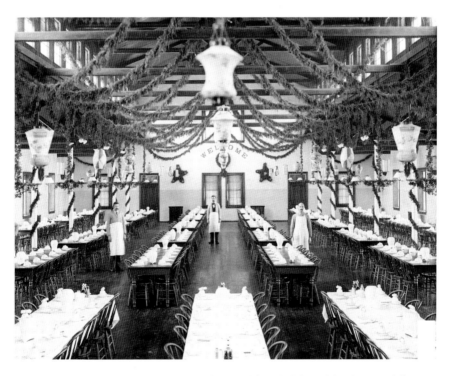

Attendants and other staff decorated the dining hall for a holiday celebration, providing a sense of festivity to the cottage-style hospital building. *Photograph, 1900, National Archives and Records Administration (418-G-33).*

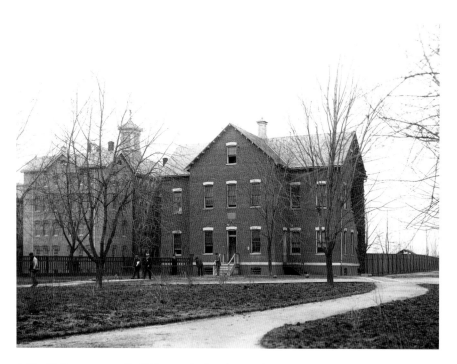

Atkins Hall, constructed in 1878, was the first Cottage Plan building at St. Elizabeths. The building was extensively altered by the addition of a third story in 1900, after this photo was taken. *Lantern slide, circa 1900, National Archives and Records Administration (418-G-25).*

funding for its construction. Alterations to Atkins Hall in 1899 included improvements to the sitting room and attendants' living spaces. As the men who lived there were to be pre-selected for their temperaments and relatively low-level symptoms, the structure did not include window bars or daytime door locks. The cottage was self-consciously designed to be homelike, notwithstanding its large size, with small-scale windows and doors.

Soon after Atkins was constructed, more cottage structures were erected nearby. Named not for dignitaries but for the sentiments they hoped to induce, the Home and Relief Buildings helped alleviate overcrowding. Both housed men; the Home building was intended for Civil War veterans and Relief for chronically ill white men. Relief had three stories, each housing patients with different diagnoses in "cheerful and airy"[25] dormitory-style rooms.

Although St. Elizabeths was a public hospital, the superintendents had the authority—and often were encouraged by Congress—to accept private, paying patients if space was available. The hospital usually could not accept

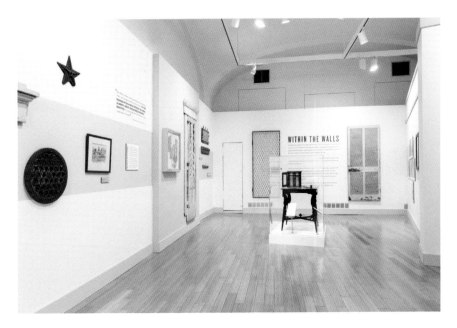

National Building Museum installation. *Photo by Yassine El Mansouri, 2017.*

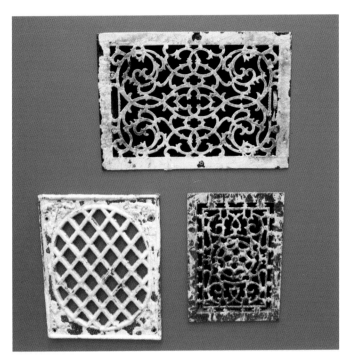

Corridors in the Center Building featured different designs on stencils, windows and ventilation grilles. *Ventilation grilles, nineteenth century, General Services Administration. NBM staff photograph, 2018.*

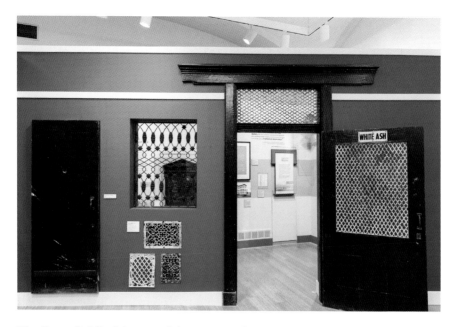

The Center Building's layout and door systems allowed for separation of patients by diagnosis, a feature fundamental to the Kirkbride Plan. *Door system, White Ash Ward, General Services Administration. Photo by Yassine El Mansouri, 2017.*

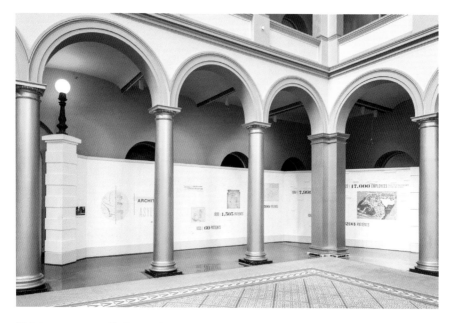

This lamppost once lit the way into the St. Elizabeths campus. It was restored to working order for the exhibition. *Gate no. 2 lamppost, early twentieth century, U.S. General Services Administration. Photo by Yassine El Mansouri, 2017.*

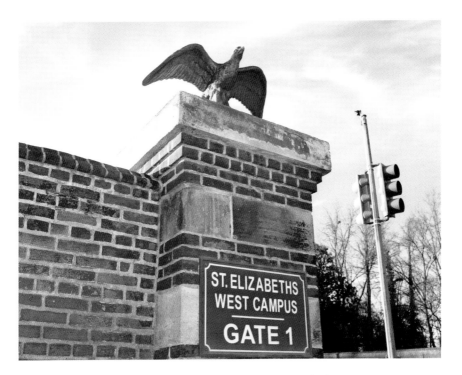

Eagle at St. Elizabeths entrance gate. *Photograph, 2017, Caitlin Bristol.*

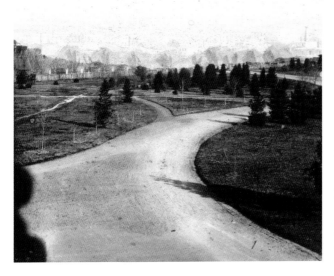

The ideal of a pastoral landscape was considered an antidote to the pressures of modern life. *Photograph, circa 1854, General Photograph Collection, Historical Society of Washington, D.C.*

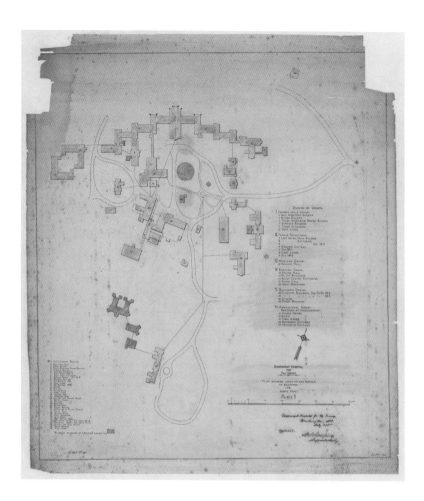

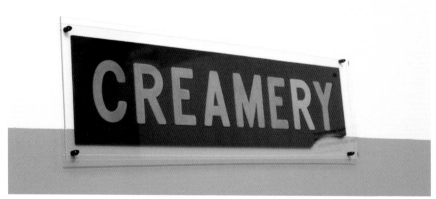

Top: Site plan, map, 1895, Library of Congress, American Architectural Foundation Collection.

Bottom: The dairy herd at St. Elizabeths provided milk for patients, served in dining halls across campus. *Creamery sign, St. Elizabeths dairy, pre-1940, U.S. General Services Administration. NBM staff photograph, 2018.*

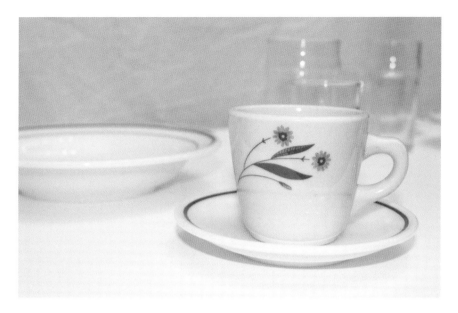

As the population grew, the design of the tableware used at St. Elizabeths changed from delicate and floral to practical, plain and institutional. *Tableware used at St. Elizabeths, twentieth century, General Services Administration. NBM staff photograph, 2018.*

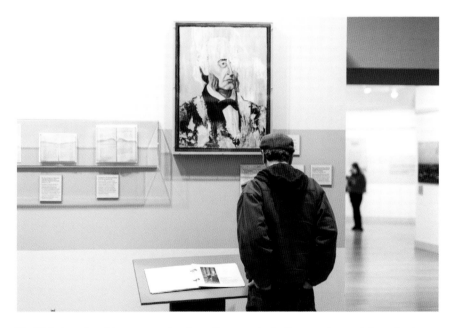

Dr. Nichols endured intense scrutiny from Congress, including two thorough investigations during his tenure at the hospital. *Painting on plaster from the Center Building, unknown artist, U.S. General Services Administration. Photo by Yassine El Mansouri, 2017.*

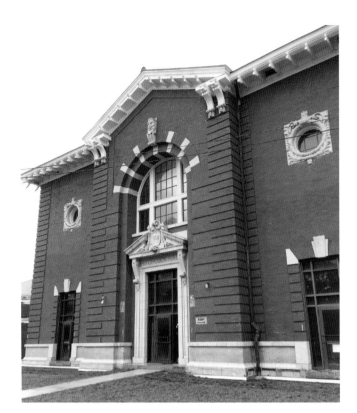

Exterior of
Hitchcock Hall.
*Photograph, 2015,
Caitlin Bristol.*

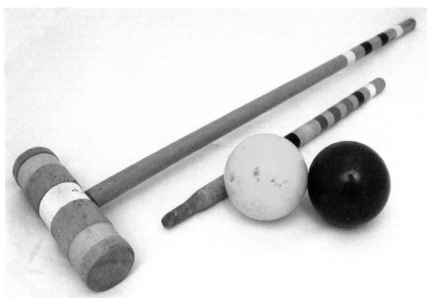

A hospital memo dated 1956 noted that most wards had their own croquet set. *Croquet set used at St. Elizabeths, twentieth century, U.S. General Services Administration. NBM staff photograph, 2018.*

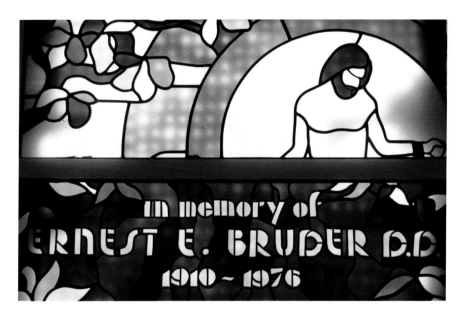

The design of this stained-glass window honored longtime chaplain Ernie Bruder, who fought for a designated building for religious services on campus. *Stained-glass window from the chapel, 1970s, St. Elizabeths Hospital Museum. NBM staff photograph, 2018.*

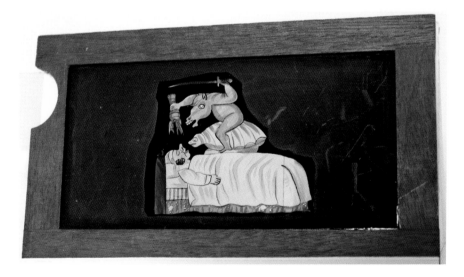

In the late nineteenth century, some doctors believed that magic lantern displays with disturbing images served a therapeutic purpose. *Magic lantern slide, manufacturer T.M. McAllister, optician, New York City, circa 1870s, U.S. National Library of Medicine. NBM staff photograph, 2018.*

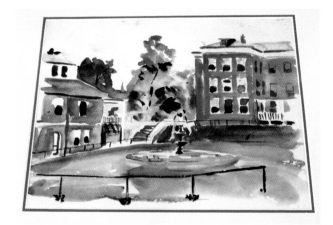

Patients' art is one way to see St. Elizabeths through the eyes of those who lived there. Art therapist Prentiss Taylor helped patients express themselves from 1943 to 1954. *Patient watercolor, National Museum of Health and Medicine. NBM staff photograph, 2018.*

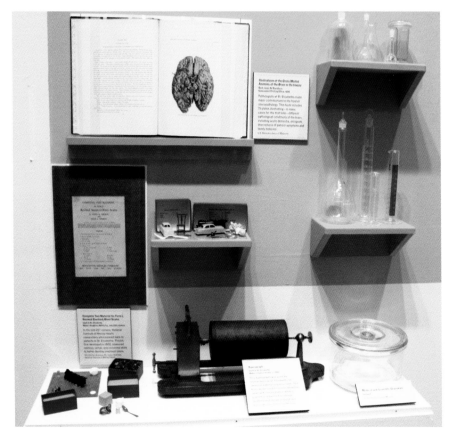

St. Elizabeths and National Institute of Mental Health researchers administered tests to patients at the hospital. *Items from various collections including National Museum of Health and Medicine; NIH Stetten Museum; Mr. Jason McEntee, National Institute of Mental Health; St. Elizabeths Hospital Museum; and U.S. National Library of Medicine. NBM staff photograph, 2018.*

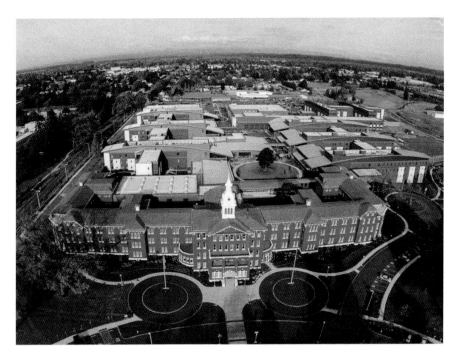

Oregon State Insane Asylum (Oregon State Hospital), Salem, Oregon. The historic 1883 building is now the Museum of Mental Health, on the campus of the Oregon State Hospital. *Photograph, 2014, Oregon State Hospital Museum of Mental Health.*

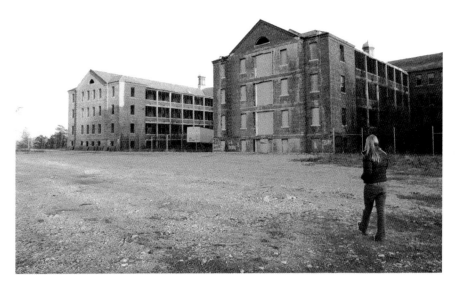

Urban explorer at Northampton State Hospital (opened 1858), Northampton, Massachusetts. *Photograph, 2007, Karan Jain, Creative Commons.*

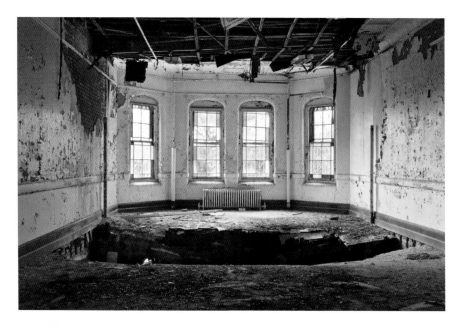

At the Hudson River State Hospital in Poughkeepsie, New York, plans to restore several of the Kirkbride buildings into residences were derailed by a 2018 arson fire. *Photograph, "Collapse, Female Ward," 2010, © Christina Tullo.*

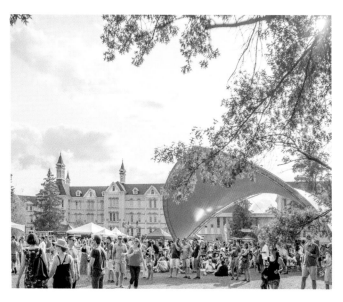

The Village at Grand Traverse Commons, Traverse City Summer Microbrew and Music Festival. *Photograph, 2015, Oden & Janelle Photography.*

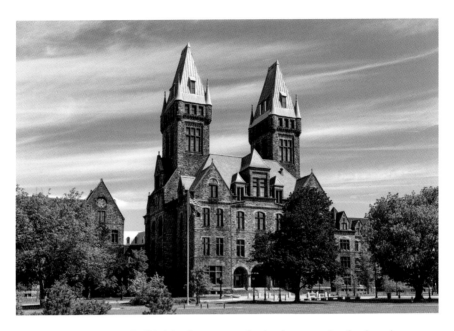

After decades of debate, Buffalo's leaders approved a development plan for the aging Kirkbride building with its iconic copper roof. After extensive renovation, the complex opened as a luxury hotel and conference center. The building shares space with the Buffalo Architecture Center. *Photograph, 2018, Joe Cascio.*

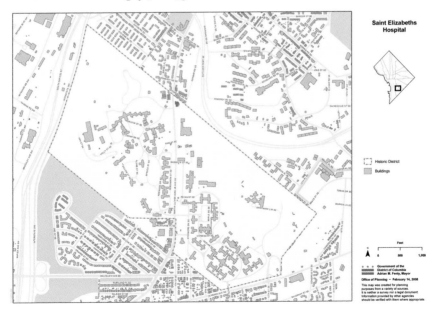

Redevelopment plans for St. Elizabeths include the reuse and restoration of most of the historic buildings on the site, which was designated a National Historic Landmark in 1991. *St. Elizabeths Historic District Map, Government of the District of Columbia, Office of Planning, 2008.*

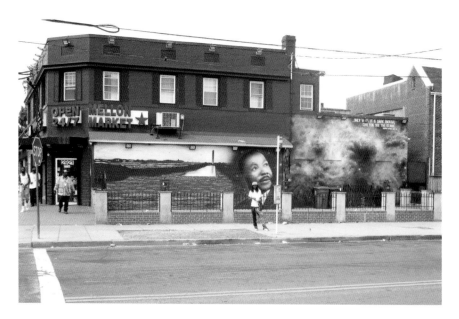

Teen photographers from the National Building Museum's Investigating Where We Live summer outreach program documented the Congress Heights neighborhood. *Photograph, 2016, Jonah Nguyen-Conyers.*

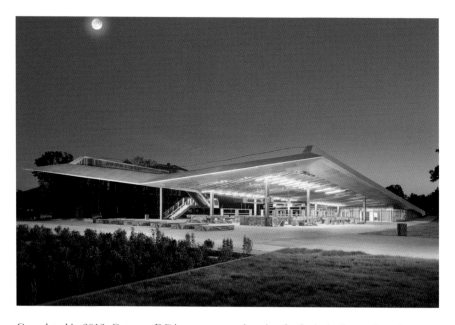

Completed in 2013, Gateway DC is a temporary location for festivals, farmers' markets, educational programing and arts events. *G8WAY DC, architect Davis Brody Bond; structural engineer Robert Silman Associates Structural Engineers, DPC, photograph, 2013, © Eric Taylor, EricTaylorPhoto.com.*

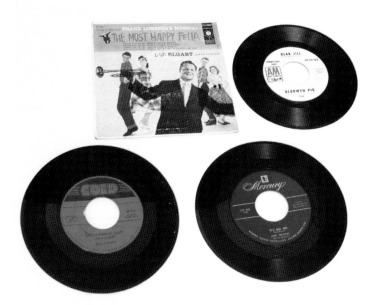

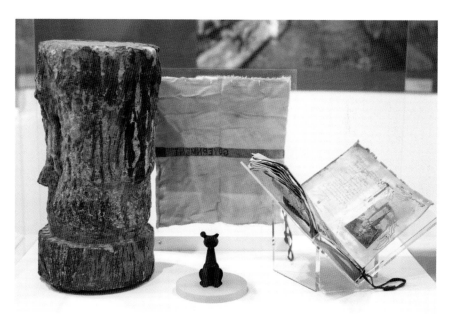

Top: These records were among the many personal materials found in the Center Building during twenty-first-century construction. *45-RPM records: "It's No Sin" (1951), "The Most Happy Fella" (1956), "Gotta Find My Baby" (1959) and "Dear Jill" (1969), found in the Center Building, U.S. General Services Administration. NBM staff photograph, 2018.*

Bottom: Items left behind in the Center Building give brief glimpses into patient life. *Patient belongings found in the Center Building, U.S. General Services Administration. Photo by Yassine El Mansouri, 2017.*

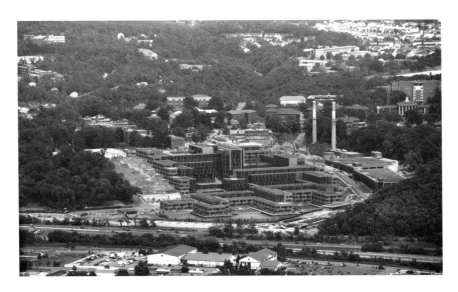

Douglas A. Munro Coast Guard Headquarters Building. *Aerial photograph, 2013,* ©
Christopher Cavas.

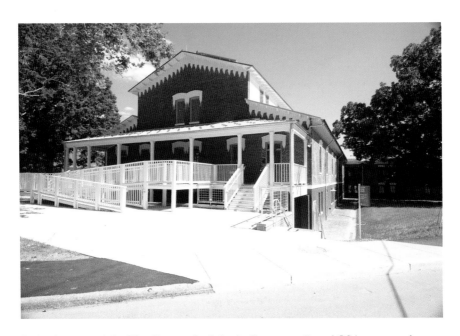

Redevelopment of the West Campus for federal office space allowed GSA to return the
1885 Dining Hall to its original use. *Photograph, 2013, U.S. General Services Administration.*

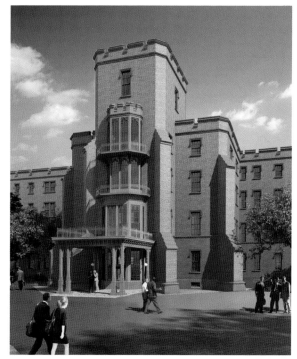

Right: This rendering shows the planned reuse of the Center Building for government offices. *Rendering, circa 2016, U.S. General Services Administration.*

Below: In 2016, contractors removed examples of flooring, decorative wall stencils, ventilation grilles and other architectural details for repair or replication and reinstallation. *Decorative wall plaster from the Center Building, U.S. General Services Administration. NBM staff photograph, 2018.*

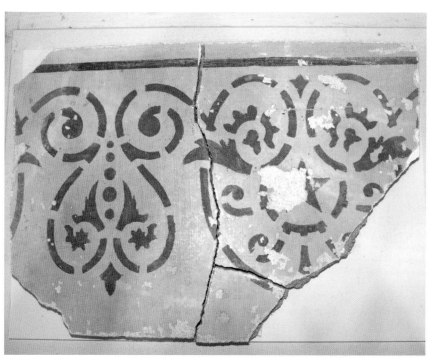

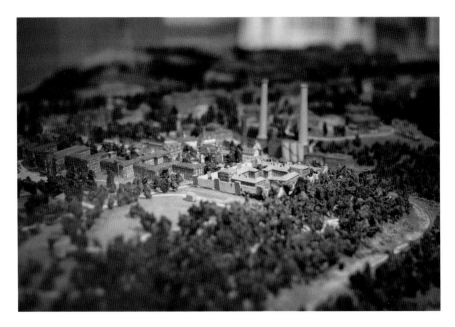

This scale model of the St. Elizabeths campus was prepared for the St. Louis World's Fair in 1904 and expanded in 1935. *Model, Center for Historic Buildings, U.S. General Services Administration. Photo by Yassine El Mansouri, 2017.*

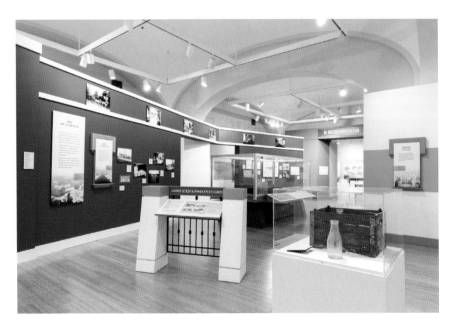

The exhibition "Architecture of an Asylum: St. Elizabeths, 1852–2017" opened at the National Building Museum in Washington, D.C., in 2017. *Photo by Yassine El Mansouri, 2017.*

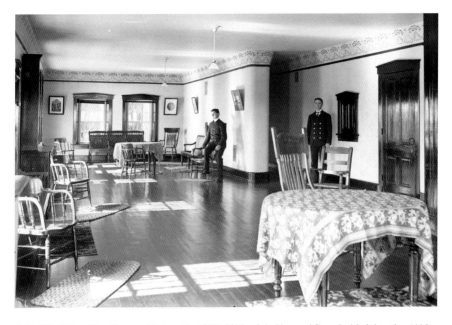

Relief Building, Day Room. *Photograph, 1905, National Archives and Records Administration (418-G-284).*

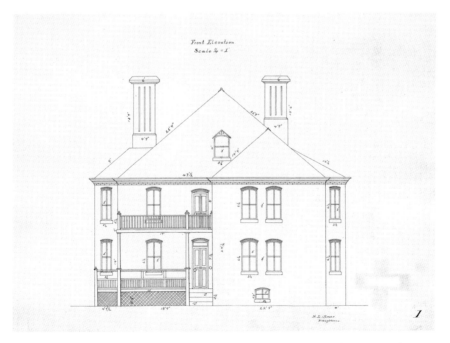

The privately funded Burroughs Cottage housed Sarah, her mother and her personal nursing staff, as well as other affluent patients. *Photograph, circa 1892, Library of Congress.*

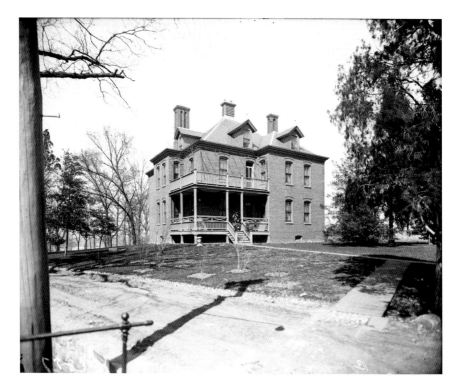

Burroughs Cottage was privately funded by the family of patient Sarah Borrows (the spelling of the building changed over time). *Photograph, 1897, National Archives and Records Administration (418-G-68).*

more men into the already crowded male wards, but this policy brought in some women as private patients. Burroughs Cottage was funded by the family of patient Sarah Borrows (the spelling of the name of the building changed over time). Completed in the 1880s, the cottage housed Sarah, her mother and her personal nursing staff. After Sarah died in 1917, the building transferred back to the hospital and was used for various purposes over time, including housing for married staff members and, much later, for the offices of a drug addiction program. Burroughs Cottage still stands as one reminder of the Cottage Plan in the architectural landscape at St. Elizabeths.

HOWARD HALL

Closing in on Maniac.[26]
—*Washington Post* headline about a St. Elizabeths escapee, 1911

In the 1880s, Congress allocated funds for Howard Hall, a new, secure building to isolate "insane criminals" of all races. Prior to this time, criminal patients had to be housed with the general population at St. Elizabeths. Increasingly, nationwide, doctors, caregivers or the courts deemed criminal patients too dangerous to be mixed with others. In addition to its primary function, however—isolating dangerous criminals—Howard Hall was used for many years as a triage area for African American men coming into the hospital, whether or not they were convicts.

Howard Hall, named for the eighteenth-century British prison reformer John Howard, included 120 single-occupancy rooms for "homicidal and dangerous" men. The original structure of Howard Hall, a quadrangle

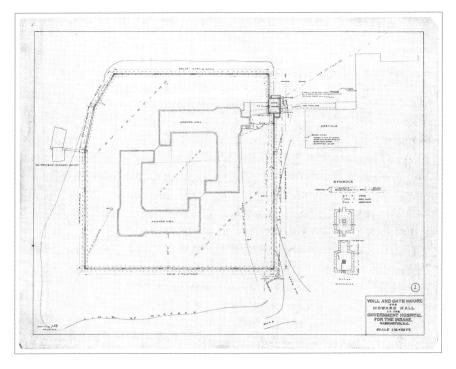

Howard Hall became overcrowded within four years and was soon expanded. Additions included new outdoor recreation space, deemed necessary by hospital officials in a 1912 report. *Drawing, 1913, Library of Congress, American Architectural Foundation Collection.*

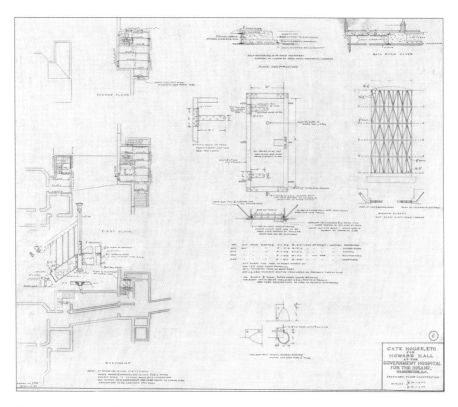

The door at Howard Hall was purposefully designed to be an extreme escape deterrent, made from a single one-inch-thick metal plate. *Drawing, 1914, Library of Congress, American Architectural Foundation Collection.*

with four wings, was completed in 1891. Howard Hall's residents could not leave the enclosed grounds; the building was completely self-contained, with its own area for field work and recreation. Convict-patients had their own schedule of religious services, outdoor activities and leisure time, separate from the rest of the patient population.

Howard Hall became overcrowded within four years. A report from the hospital administration to the Department of the Interior requested funding for a new perimeter wall for Howard Hall, noting, "It is impossible to maintain desperate criminals in security when the windows offer such easy communication between the outside world and the interior of the building."[27] The wall would provide security as well as new outdoor recreation space, deemed necessary by hospital officials in a 1912 report, as the "courtyard is stifling hot and almost uninhabitable in the summer time."[28] Security was a top priority in the design of Howard Hall due to a consistent problem with

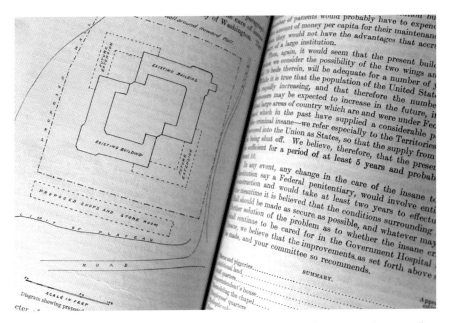

This report to the Department of the Interior requested funding for a new perimeter wall for Howard Hall. *From* Needs of Government Hospital for the Insane, *report, Isaac Blackburn, 1911, U.S. National Library of Medicine. NBM staff photograph, 2018.*

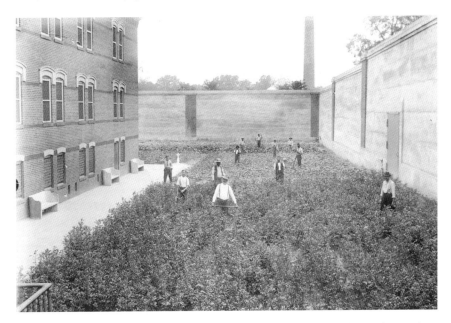

Howard Hall was completely self-contained, with its own area for gardening and recreation. A 1915 addition of a twenty-four-foot surrounding wall provided extra outdoor space and security. *Photograph, 1916, National Archives and Records Administration (418-G-153).*

escapes. The building's iron doors were purposefully designed as an escape deterrent, with a one-inch-thick metal plate. Still, local newspapers often printed salacious reports of St. Elizabeths escapes, including one involving a group of five patients in 1911. It took three years to secure the funding and complete, but in 1915, the new twenty-four-foot surrounding wall began to provide extra outdoor space for Howard Hall residents.

In use for more than six decades, Howard Hall was demolished in the 1950s and replaced by a utilitarian patient dormitory building also named after the prison reformer. Built in 1959, the John Howard Pavilion for the Criminally Insane was, in turn, demolished in 2010 and replaced by a new hospital on the East Campus. Today, forensic patients, as "insane criminals" are now known, live in the same hospital building as civil admissions, just as they once did in the mid-1800s, albeit with more sophisticated and rigid isolation from the general population.

GODDING'S EXPANSION

Howard Hall and the hospital's Cottage Plan buildings—Relief, Home and Atkins—successfully segregated patients by race, diagnosis or criminal status. The practice of constructing smaller, specialized buildings continued under Superintendent Godding with the Dix, Toner, Oaks and Allison Buildings.

Named for hospital founder and activist Dorothea Dix, Dix Buildings 1 through 3 (Willow, Linden and Holly) made up part of Superintendent Godding's expansion and specialization plan. Dix 1 and 2 housed white women suffering from epilepsy. Dix 3 housed African American women with the same disorder. The Toner Building, an infirmary, opened in 1890 on what had once been farmland. The structure, built some distance from the Center Building for relative seclusion on a busy campus, included large windows and outdoor exercise space. It was named after J.M. Toner, a prominent local physician and the president of the hospital's board of visitors. The Oaks dormitories were originally built for white men with epilepsy and later housed African American women. Built on land that had been previously used for farming, the Oaks Buildings provided some separation and quiet for patients.

The four-building Allison group for white soldiers and sailors formed the last of Superintendent Godding's cottage-style expansion in the 1890s. Architectural differences for bedridden veterans included open sleeping

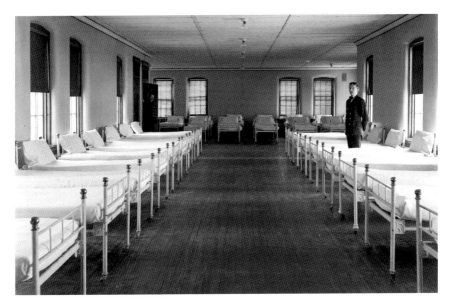

The Oaks Buildings provided separate, quiet lodging for epileptic, white male patients as part of the 1890s expansion. *Photograph, circa 1905, National Archives and Records Administration (418-G-203).*

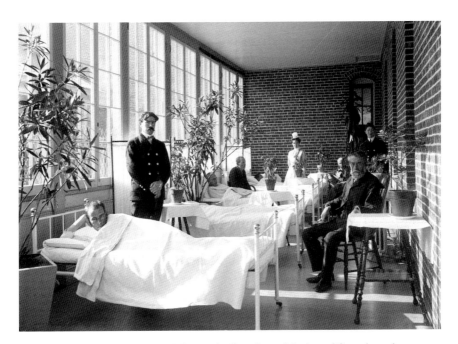

The Allison Buildings for white soldiers and sailors formed the last of Superintendent Godding's expansion in the 1890s. *Photograph, 1910, National Archives and Records Administration (418-G-15).*

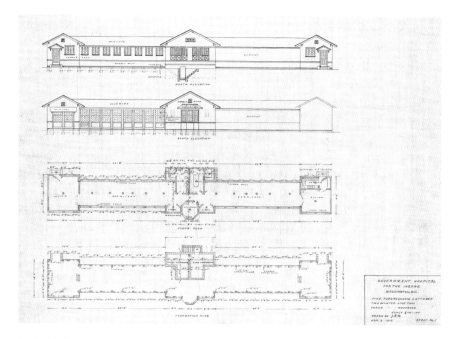

By 1914, five cottages were housing twenty tuberculosis patients each. *Drawing, 1913, Library of Congress, American Architectural Foundation Collection.*

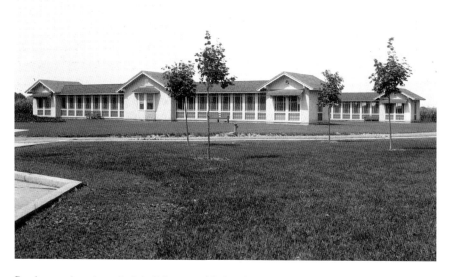

Porches on the tuberculosis buildings provided patients with fresh air and sunlight, both thought to be curatives for the disease. *Photograph, circa 1916, National Archives and Records Administration (418-G-311).*

porches, as well as doorways designed to be wide enough to allow movement of beds on casters. However, the Allison Building sleeping porches were enclosed in the 1930s to fulfill demand for more year-round sleeping, dining and recreation space.

Early in the twentieth century, with tuberculosis rampant in the general population and at the hospital, five new cottages (three for men, two for women) housed twenty TB patients each. Porches on these buildings provided patients with fresh air and sunlight, both thought to be curatives for the disease. The cottages were later demolished, and a larger, permanent building for TB patients was built in 1931. With the widespread use of antibiotics mostly eradicating the disease, the Permanent Tuberculosis Building was later repurposed as the Behavioral Sciences Building.

THE RICHARDSON GROUP

St. Elizabeths' third superintendent, Alonzo Richardson, renewed a program of large-scale new construction on the campus, although he did not live to see it come to fruition. Richardson began the development of a new plan for a series of buildings on both the older West Campus and the East Campus, which had to date been used primarily for farming. The work was completed by the next superintendent, William White.

Prominent landscape architect Frederick Law Olmsted visited the campus in 1901 and promoted an organized growth plan. "Present grounds are much cluttered and confused in arrangement not only of buildings but of trees, shrubs, roads, paths, etc.," he wrote. "Buildings are too closely arranged for proper segregation of different classes of patients."[29] Most of Olmsted's plans were never implemented; however, Superintendent White later took some of his suggestions, including moving buildings to better organize operations. For example, in 1905, the Rest Building (the mortuary) was moved to make more space for the laboratory. But Olmsted's underlying point—that the campus was an old-fashioned array of buildings without an organized plan—stuck with Superintendent Richardson. He began a major expansion, which was completed after his death, with a design competition. Only a few decades after adopting the Cottage Plan, St. Elizabeths had officially left it far behind.

The Boston architectural firm Shepley, Rutan & Coolidge won the contest for a $900,000 federal government appropriation to design a

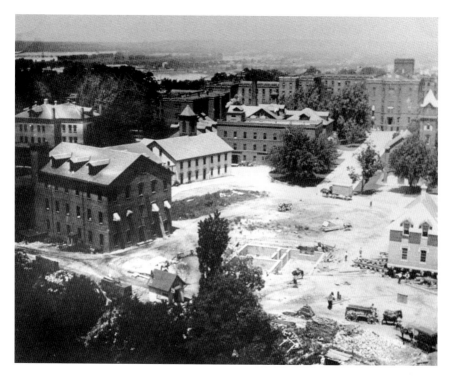

Above: In 1905, the Rest Building (the mortuary) was moved to make more space for a new laboratory. *Photograph, 1905, U.S. National Library of Medicine.*

Opposite, top: Superintendent Richardson began major construction on the campus in 1900. This new construction emphasized a single architectural aesthetic for the site. *Map, 1908, Library of Congress, American Architectural Foundation Collection.*

Opposite, bottom: By the early twentieth century, most patients ate in segregated communal dining halls throughout campus, including the African American Dining Hall in Building Q. *Photograph, circa 1915, National Archives and Records Administration (418-P-348).*

staggering number of new buildings: fifteen new structures for patients and administrative offices. The new construction followed one cohesive design to emphasize a single architectural aesthetic for the site.

The winning design was influenced by the City Beautiful movement, an urban planning philosophy popular at the time that emphasized the monumental grandeur of Neoclassical style within a landscaped setting. The new buildings—identified simply by letters rather than names of local or national dignitaries, provided space for one thousand patients as well as kitchens, dining rooms and support services. The wards featured areas for sitting, dormitory-style sleeping and extra space for temporary isolation. The

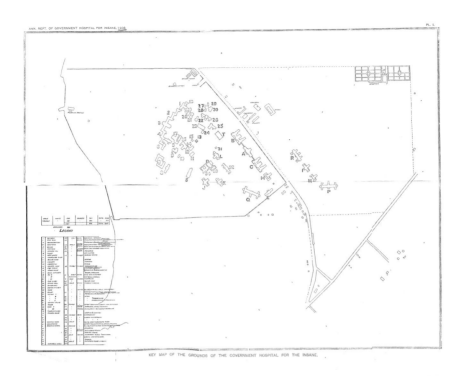

KEY MAP OF THE GROUNDS OF THE GOVERNMENT HOSPITAL FOR THE INSANE.

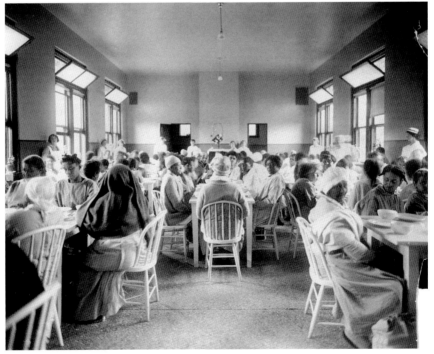

buildings had arched windows, prominently detailed entranceways, red-tiled roofs and high ceilings. In contrast to the Victorian-era cottages on campus, the letter buildings were constructed in the monumental Renaissance Revival style, with an institutional feel—large buildings in red brick with limestone detailing and tile roofs, for a distinctly modern and formal look to welcome the new century.

Richardson's letter buildings were built in stages, for different purposes. The first of these were constructed along Nichols Avenue, inside the stone wall on the West Campus. Building A, or the Administration Building, featured grand white limestone columns conveying the dignity of the federal institution and was flanked by Buildings B and C. The Administration Building housed medical staff as well as offices and included a medical library. Buildings B and C were used for male and female admitting wards so that proper assessments could be made before placing patients in appropriate buildings and particular wards. These buildings had hydrotherapy units in the basement, enclosed porches, a surgical department and single rooms.

Other letter buildings housed white soldiers and sailors transferred from the National Home for Disabled Volunteer Soldiers. Physicians also resided in some of the buildings. Building E was the nurses' home; Buildings J and K

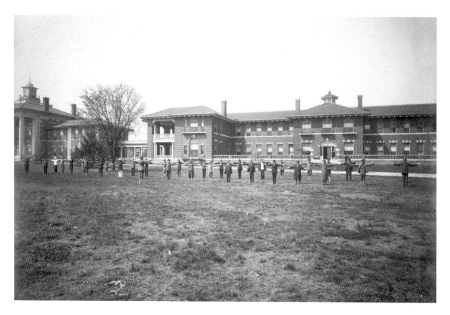

The new buildings' Renaissance Revival institution style brought a more modern look to campus. *Photograph, 1918, National Archives and Records Administration (418-G-343).*

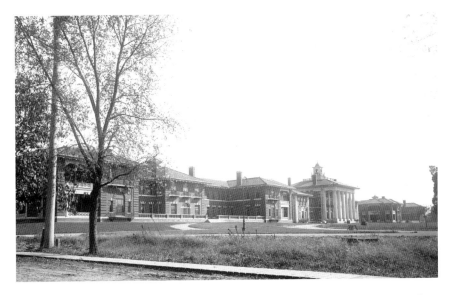

A, B and C Buildings were part of Richardson's "letter building" expansion plan, providing space for one thousand patients as well as kitchens, dining rooms and support services. *Lantern slide, National Archives and Records Administration (418-G-5).*

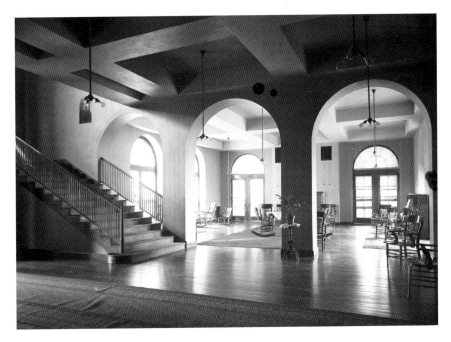

The L Building was part of the Shepley, Rutan & Coolidge expansion. *Photograph, 1905, National Archives and Records Administration (418-G-183).*

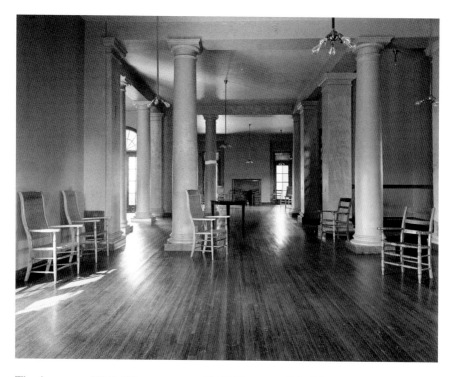

The day room of N Building, constructed in 1902 as part of the Richardson expansion on the East Campus, featured open space and formal columns. *Photograph, 1905, National Archives and Records Administration (418-G-197).*

were for African American female patients; Building L was for white female patients; and Building Q was a receiving ward for female patients, with a hydrotherapy section.

The next stage of letters, across Nichols Avenue on the East Campus, included Buildings I, N, P and R. These were the first patient wards on the East Campus and housed some of the most "disturbed" patients on the site. Building I was for "infirm, untidy" white women; Building N housed "epileptic and feebleminded" white women; Building P provided wards for white and African American female patients; and Building R included mixed wards. They were purposefully set back from the road so as to maintain privacy for the patients.

Significantly, the Richardson Group marked the first time patient facilities spread across Nichols Avenue. Up to that point, the almost two-hundred-acre East Campus had been used entirely for food production for the hospital and for staff cottages. The underpass constructed in

1903 below Nichols Avenue signaled a vast expansion of the hospital's population and scope and brought patients, staff and carriages more easily to the new buildings. And in the next wave of East Campus construction, the tunnel was expanded in 1938 to accommodate automobile traffic in addition to pedestrians and horses. By 1940, there was almost an even distribution of buildings on both sides of Nichols Avenue.

MID-TWENTIETH-CENTURY EXPANSION

A third period of major growth took place in the 1920s and 1930s under St. Elizabeths' fourth superintendent, William White, and included new patient buildings set in orderly quadrangles. Maple Quadrangle and the Continuous Treatment buildings on the East Campus took over the remainder of what had been the hospital's working farmland. Most of this construction was in the Italian Renaissance Revival style, characterized here by red-tiled roofs, large arched entrances and overhanging eaves. The imposing structures have cupolas and stone balustrades, as well as enclosed porches with large screened windows. An exception is the 1924 Glenside building, a one-story masonry structure built for geriatric patients that did not conform to the other buildings stylistically.

The arrangement and siting of the Maple Quadrangle was part of a larger nationwide emphasis on orderly campus landscape architecture. The buildings represented a shift in treatment philosophy at the hospital as well, with an emphasis on acute care for patients who could recover quickly and be discharged. The Maple Quadrangle was built in a similar Italian Renaissance Revival style as the Richardson Group, albeit at a larger scale. The new group included five- and six-story red brick structures with limestone detailing and tile roofs, constructed in a formal plan around a central quadrangle. The Medical Sciences Building opened as a general hospital for the campus, designed by architect L.H. Dittrich. The Male Receiving Building (White Building) opened in 1934, and the women's counterpart (Nichols Building) opened in 1936. Both were named after superintendents of the hospital and held several hundred acute, or temporary, patients.

The Continuous Treatment complex, conversely, was built to house chronic patients. These eight buildings added hundreds of beds to the campus in the 1930s and 1940s. The CT cluster reflected a new understanding about the role of the hospital in providing long-term, probably lifetime, care. The

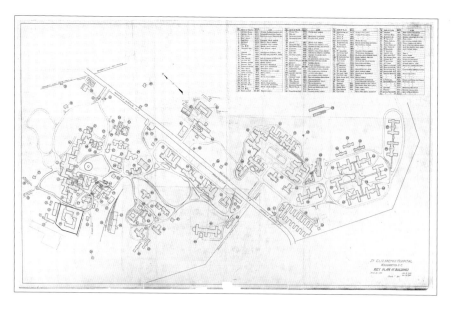

By 1940, major expansion was almost over. Subsequent buildings included the large complexes on the East Campus. *Map, 1940, Library of Congress, American Architectural Foundation Collection.*

buildings sat in an oval configuration, with a central kitchen and dining facility in the center.

Changes were afoot all over the campus as the population surged. Aging infrastructure on the historic West Campus led Congress to appropriate funds to tear down older buildings—the Toner and Oaks structures—in favor of new construction on the East Campus. In replacing the older, smaller, more ornate structures with utilitarian buildings, St. Elizabeths' leaders finally and totally abandoned the nineteenth-century belief in an architectural cure for mental illness. The very tenets of moral treatment and guidelines of Thomas Kirkbride, in which one stately, ornate building could provide solace for a small number of patients, gave way to the realities of a modern mental health crisis.

The final period of growth at St. Elizabeths occurred with peak population in the mid-twentieth century, under the leadership of the hospital's fifth superintendent, Winfred Overholser. To accommodate the specialized needs of such a busy, working campus, new buildings in midcentury included living accommodations for staff as well as patients on both sides of Nichols Avenue. On the East Campus, two-story Barton Hall, a new home for nurses, was built in the Colonial Revival style, with a wood portico and simple detailing in contrast to the Renaissance Revival structures nearby. On the West Campus, Hagan Hall replaced the American Red Cross building as an entertainment venue after a destructive fire in 1942.

Three major patient buildings were constructed in this period in a loosely modernist style, each with multistory wards housing hundreds of patients. The new buildings did not share architectural vocabulary with the older structures, other than red-colored bricks, nor were they sited in relation to existing buildings. Haydon Hall, a five-story building dating from 1952 in the modern style, housed geriatric, chronic patients. The building was named after Edith Haydon, the director of nursing at the hospital from the 1920s through the 1950s. The Dorothea Dix Pavilion and the John Howard Pavilion, respectively built in 1956 and 1959, were multistory buildings that housed hundreds of patients. Howard Pavilion replaced the aging Howard Hall for forensic patients, retaining only the name. Dix Pavilion, named after the nineteenth-

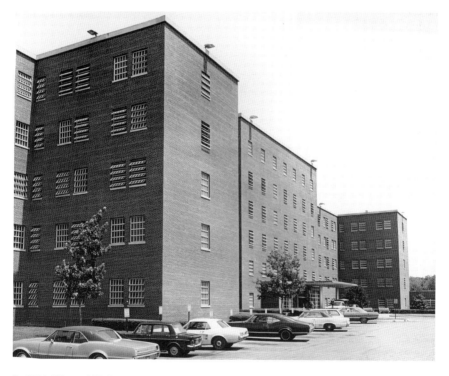

In 1959, Howard Hall was demolished and patients moved into the new, larger, John Howard Pavilion for the Criminally Insane, which lasted half a century until being demolished in 2010. *Photograph, circa 1960s, National Archives and Records Administration (418 STE-132).*

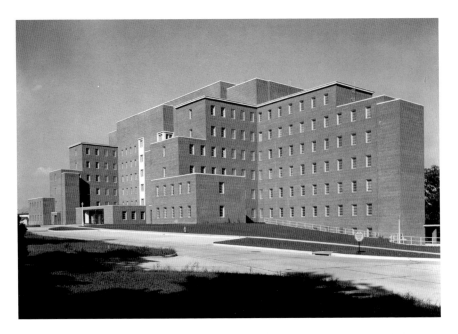

The ten-story Dorothea Dix Pavilion was built in 1956 for 420 patients. *Photograph, circa 1960, National Archives and Records Administration (418 HB-11-1).*

century activist who helped found the hospital, was a ten-story structure built over a filled-in ravine and used for new admissions and acute care. The final major patient building of the twentieth century was the Rehabilitation Medicine Building, constructed in the modernist style in 1963. Patients lived in all these buildings until they were finally emptied, and mostly demolished, after the new hospital opened on the East Campus in 2010.

PART IV
LIFE AT ST. ELIZABETHS

RACIAL SEGREGATION

Opinion and practice vary somewhat in regard to the propriety of associating white and colored insane persons in the same wards of the same institution; but I believe the majority of practical men decidedly condemn such association, and resort to it, if at all, only as a choice of great evils.[30]
—Superintendent Charles Nichols,
Report to the Secretary of the Interior, 1854

Many mental health hospitals in America were racially segregated until the 1950s. Some states built entirely separate hospitals for African Americans, such as Virginia's Central Lunatic Asylum for the Colored Insane, founded in 1869. St. Elizabeths always admitted African American patients, yet the campus was segregated by race until federal desegregation in 1954. Other nonwhite patients, although such populations were low, lived in either white or African American wards at the administration's discretion. At a time when architecture was considered part of the treatment, patients of color generally experienced both inferior quality of care and inferior living conditions while at the hospital. Gay and lesbian patients also experienced prejudicial treatment, but they do not seem to have experienced architectural segregation.

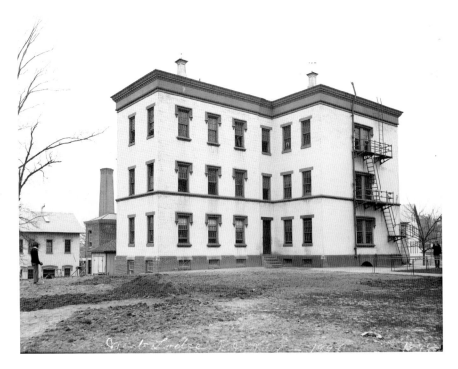

Originally built in 1860 for African American men, the West Lodge was expanded thirty years later. *Photograph, 1898, National Archives and Records Administration (418-G-331).*

St. Elizabeths' first African American patients, some of whom may have been formerly enslaved, lived in a "colored wing" of the Center Building until Congress appropriated funds for separate residence halls. Like the city at large, racial boundaries became porous at St. Elizabeths during the Civil War. Racial segregation became impossible to maintain in practice due to an enlarged population and altered racial demographics. For example, the navy commandeered the residence building intended for African American men. Non-military patients were relocated wherever possible.

The first buildings constructed specifically for African American patients were among the first buildings on the campus: the East and West Lodges. Superintendent Nichols specified that the lodges should be "not less than 200 nor more than 400 feet"[31] from the Center Building. In 1900, the board of visitors recommended moving black patients completely across Nichols Avenue to emphasize segregation. That never came to pass, but segregation was stark in any case. The lodges "for the colored insane" sat behind the Center Building and overlooked stables and service buildings rather than

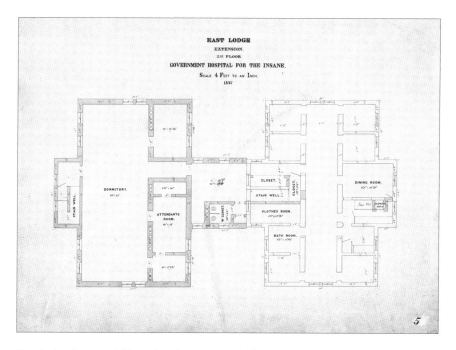

East Lodge, home to African American women, had an open dormitory for patients. Most white patients in the Center Building lived in individual rooms. *Drawing, 1887, Library of Congress, American Architectural Foundation Collection.*

the bucolic river view. The buildings also had significant architectural differences. Most white patients in the Center Building lived in individual rooms, according to Kirkbride's guidelines; the West Lodge for men and the East Lodge for women instead provided only open dormitories for patients.

In the nineteenth century, with military veterans from across the country making up at least half of the patient population, black patients often arrived after being transferred from Washington Asylum Hospital (later known as Gallinger Municipal Hospital and then D.C. General). Once they got to St. Elizabeths, they lived in lesser facilities with smaller rooms than the white patients and did not have the opportunity to take advantage of new treatment innovations. Recreational activities, when offered to both races, were often held separately or on different days. Organizations that visited campus sponsored segregated events and occasionally offered entertainment such as vaudeville acts with performers in blackface. Well into the twentieth century, treatment, work and entertainment at the hospital remained segregated and often inferior for nonwhite patients.

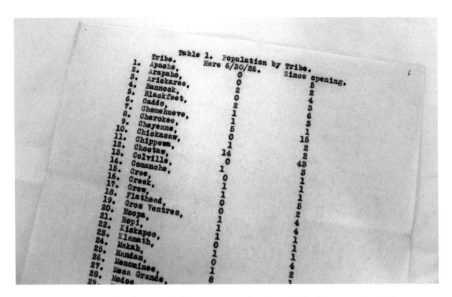

The environment at the Canton Asylum was notoriously terrible. However, in 1926, Superintendent H.R. Hummer, who had previously worked at St. Elizabeths, filed a positive report. *From* Annual Report and Census to the U.S. Department of the Interior, Indian Field Service, Canton Asylum for Insane Indians, 1926, *U.S. National Library of Medicine. NBM staff photograph, 2018.*

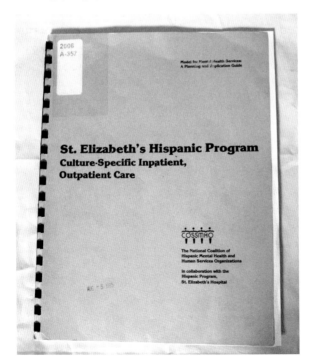

This report outlined guidelines for working with the hospital's four hundred Hispanic patients. *From* St. Elizabeths Hispanic Program: Culture-Specific Inpatient, Outpatient Care Report, *circa 1980, U.S. National Library of Medicine. NBM staff photograph, 2018.*

Racial segregation and discrimination informed staff experience as well; throughout the hospital attendants and nurses remained exclusively white until 1937, and doctors until 1954.

As the nation's only federally funded mental health hospital, St. Elizabeths admitted Native Americans from federal reservations, but only a handful at any given time. South Dakota's Canton (Hiawatha) Asylum for Insane Indians took over this role when it opened in 1902. After an investigation, however, the Department of the Interior's Bureau of Indian Affairs cited abuses and indicated that most of the patients exhibited no signs of mental illness. In 1933, the government closed the hospital, sending most patients home. The sixty-nine remaining patients who were determined to have a true mental health diagnosis came to St. Elizabeths. The men were housed in a separate ward, while the few women lived with the white women. Many of the patients stayed the rest of their lives in Washington; fourteen are buried in the cemetery.

Throughout its history, St. Elizabeths housed patients of all races, finally desegregating all the wards in the 1950s. By the 1980s, with a growing population of Latino residents, a special report outlined guidelines for working with the hospital's four hundred such patients—revealing limited knowledge of cultural differences yet promoting some sensitivity. Recommendations included hanging "brightly colored paintings," playing Spanish-language music and introducing "culture-specific psychodrama," among other supportive activities. The idea was that doing so would alleviate the patients' "sense of separation, alienation, and marginality."[32]

SELF-SUFFICIENCY AND FARMING

[It is] *the obvious duty of those having the care of indigent insane, for whom provision is made at the public expense, to make them self-supporting.*[33]
—Superintendent Charles Nichols

St. Elizabeths, like many other such institutions, provided much of its own food and support services in the nineteenth and early twentieth centuries. While never completely self-sufficient, the hospital supplied energy and water instead of relying on city utilities and furnished raw materials and labor for daily functions. Staff purchased some finished goods in town—such as tools, overcoats and slippers—while store-bought supplies like nails, seeds and fabric were used to produce clothing, plant crops and build other goods. A proprietary rail system brought goods and raw materials to the site. Train tracks required frequent repairs, with a complete overhaul in 1935. The hospital even had its own railcar. Saint Elizabeth No. 4, known as "Little Lizzie," was built in 1950 by the H.K. Porter Company and was the last locomotive to transport coal on the hospital's dedicated spur of the Baltimore & Ohio Rail line.

To get all this work done, the hospital employed hundreds of laborers and farmers, many from the surrounding Washington neighborhoods. The hospital also relied on patient labor in its early years. In fact, at the turn of the twentieth century, prevailing medical beliefs identified productive work not as exploitative for patients but rather as an important part of the therapy program. Patients—up to a quarter of the total population during the last decades of the nineteenth century and 40 percent by the 1920s—worked on the campus. They raked the vast lawns, cared for crops and other plantings in gardens and greenhouses and supported infrastructure projects

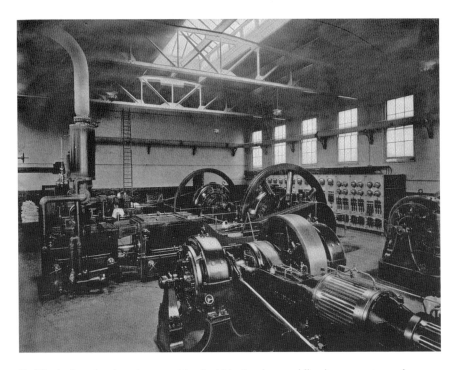

St. Elizabeths existed as almost an island within the city, providing its own water and power. *Engine room of the power house of the U.S. Hospital for the Insane, Thomas W. Power Engineering Company, circa 1907, Historical Society of Washington, D.C., General Photograph Collection.*

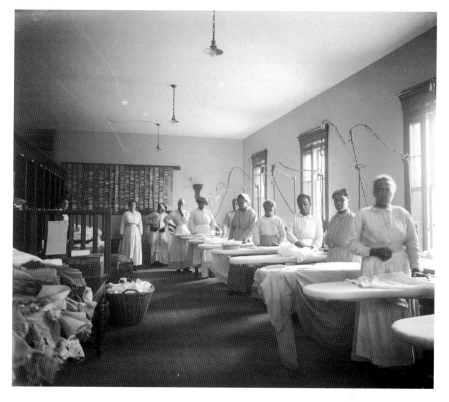

Work in the laundry was often considered part of a therapy program. *Photograph, 1918, National Archives and Records Administration (418-G-188).*

through light construction and excavation for new roads and buildings. Patients' individual job assignments differed based on their diagnoses, as well as race, age and gender. More black men were assigned to manual labor on the campus, for example, whereas white patients had opportunities to work as carpenters, tailors and seamstresses. White women were more often tasked with indoor occupations in their own wards or buildings, such as sewing, while black women might be assigned heavy laundry labor. Overall, white men were given a far wider range of tasks on the grounds, farms and industrial shops.

Using tracks built into the basement floor, workers transported sheets, towels and clothing across the vast length of the Center Building. In 1896, Superintendent Godding oversaw construction of a new facility to process more than fifty thousand pieces of laundry per week. The new wash house contained a machine and hand tubs room, a drying room, an ironing room,

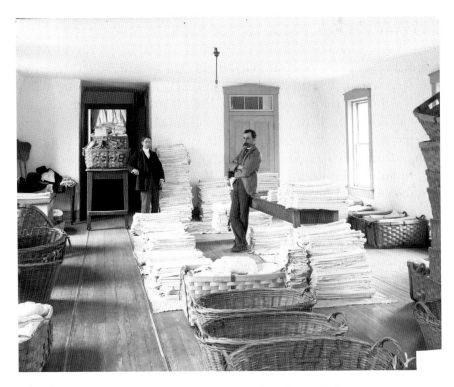

In 1896, Superintendent Godding oversaw construction of a new facility to process more than fifty thousand pieces of laundry per week. *Photograph, 1897, National Archives and Records Administration (418-G-186).*

an airing room, a yard with soaking tubs and a room for making soap. Patients also worked in shops making furniture, wooden hangers, mattresses and clothing.

Farming was perhaps the most important outlet for patient labor, as well as a constant need on the campus. Many nineteenth-century patients, especially men, had once worked as farmhands, so they arrived at the hospital with skills and comfort around animals and agriculture. Given the size of the patient and staff population, in many ways St. Elizabeths had no choice but to provide much of its own food. Nineteenth-century Washington did not have markets that would have sold enough food in bulk quantities to feed such a large community. In annual reports and testimony to Congress, the hospital administration detailed its production of fruit, vegetables and animal products for consumption. Patients and staff farmed grains such as hay, oats and rye, as well as several varieties of grapes and other fruits, and bottled milk in St. Elizabeths' own creamery.

In 1869, St. Elizabeths purchased a large tract for farming, close to 150 acres. This land, adjacent to the site across Nichols Avenue, became the East Campus. Soon, new construction included barns, farmworkers' cottages and feed storage structures. The farmhouses were typically vernacular-style wood-frame construction, making them instantly discernable from the hospital wards. Similarly, the dry barn was constructed as a typical mid-Atlantic vernacular dairy barn. Although patients worked on the farm for both practical and therapeutic reasons, the hospital also employed a large staff of farmworkers.

Although the farms remained active in the life of the hospital, after 1900, farming was increasingly consolidated elsewhere, using hired staff rather than patient labor. More and more, farmland on the East Campus was taken over by hospital buildings. In the 1890s, St. Elizabeths expanded yet again by purchasing adjacent farmland, the former Shepherd Farm, and Superintendent Godding convinced Congress to purchase four hundred acres at the Oxon Hill Farm in nearby Prince Georges County, Maryland. At the height of farm production on the campus, in the 1890s, the hospital

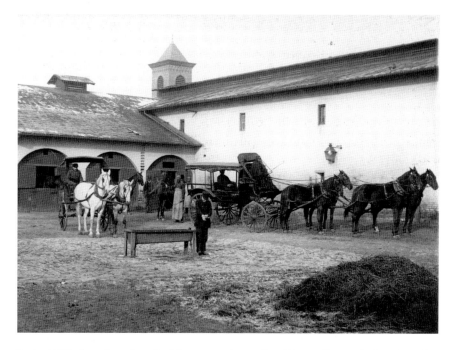

In the 1880s, Superintendent Godding wrote about a "world apart," an agricultural utopia in which patients would live in farmhouses, work with animals and cultivate the land. *Photograph, nineteenth century, National Archives and Records Administration (418-P-564).*

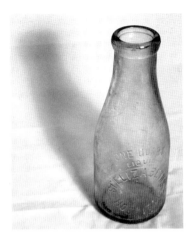

Milk production remained in operation at the farm at St. Elizabeths through the mid-twentieth century. *Milk bottles, pre-1940s, General Services Administration. NBM staff photograph, 2018.*

supervised a total of eight hundred acres of land, of which six hundred acres was used for agriculture.

Despite the success and growth of the farming program, serving food in dozens of locations, to thousands of people, several times each day was a constant concern of the hospital administration. Complaints were often leveled as to the quality of the food, beginning with early investigations of Superintendent Nichols and continuing for the next century. In a 1906 investigation of Superintendent White, for example, the staff charged that "food [was] not palatable and exceedingly unwholesome."[34] For the most part, the board of visitors and Congress dismissed these concerns.

By the 1920s, the focus of the farming program shifted from providing food for patients to feeding the dairy herds. Milk production remained in operation through the mid-twentieth century. The piggeries—which housed six hundred pigs and included yards, fattening pens, farrowing pens, bedding, a garbage area and a slaughterhouse—remained even longer. However, a new law regulating feed for pigs in Maryland affected these operations and led to the complete sell-off of the animals by 1948. In 1959, the Oxon Hill Farm, then known as Godding Croft, ceased production for the hospital. Finally, after 110 years of farming, all food production at St. Elizabeths came to an end. Even when bulk groceries were purchased elsewhere, however, cooking for thousands of patients still provided jobs for many local employees.

Water supply, in addition to food production, was also a constant problem for the hospital. Tapping springs for drinking water and relying on the Anacostia River for other uses—laundry, housekeeping—was sufficient for a while, but even though wells provided up to five thousand gallons per day, the demand for water kept growing. Most of Washington was covered by a public water system, but the thousands of residents at St. Elizabeths still relied on the increasingly polluted Anacostia River. Teams of wagons transported the water from the river to the hospital. In the 1880s, additional wells were dug and connected to a pumping station, providing water pressure for the Center

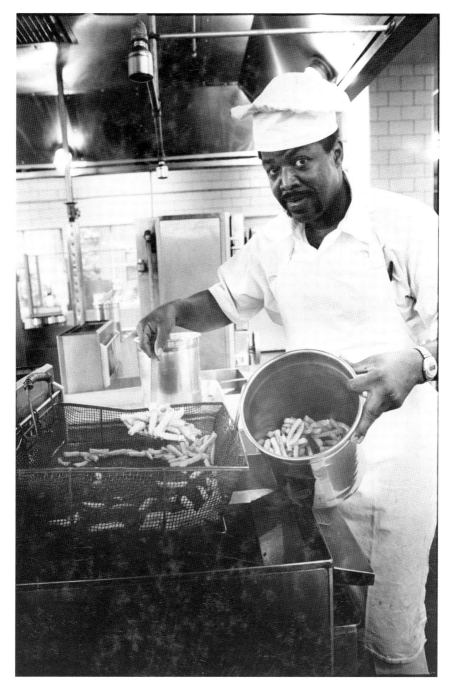

Chefs worked throughout campus preparing food for thousands of people every day.
Photograph, circa 1980s, National Museum of Health and Medicine.

Building, with tanks in the attic to store the river water. Water contamination was found to be the cause of several typhoid outbreaks in the early twentieth century, as the kitchens diluted condensed milk with hydrant water. Once the source of the problem was identified, the disease was contained. The wells and ravines were filled when the grounds were leveled in the 1960s. Water has continued to be a major concern on the campus; the water tower at St. Elizabeths has long been a source of neighborhood derision, providing only weak water pressure to nearby residents. Recent developments at the site will bring improvements to the wider community, as DC Water finally replaced the aging water tower in 2018.

HOSPITAL LEADERSHIP AND STAFF

I feel as if I was living over a volcano all the time.[35]

—Charles Nichols, 1869

Five superintendents served St. Elizabeths during its first century. All leaders in the national mental health field, these men helped to enshrine St. Elizabeths' reputation as a model of government-sponsored healthcare. The hospital's first five superintendents all lived at the Center Building, following Kirkbride's guidelines from the 1850s. The décor and architectural embellishments in the superintendent's office and living quarters reflected the prestige befitting the leader of a federal hospital. From Charles Nichols, who opened the hospital in 1855, to Winfred Overholser, who retired in 1962, the first five superintendents saw the hospital through constant population growth, ceaseless construction projects and periodic controversy. Superintendent Overholser's departure in 1962 marked the beginning of a new era of modern management, as he was the last hospital leader to live at the site.

St. Elizabeths' early superintendents submitted annual reports to a prestigious board of visitors. The first such committee included mental health reformer Dorothea Dix, Secretary of the Smithsonian Institution Joseph Henry and the surgeons general of the army and the navy. The board of visitors outlined the rules and regulations for the superintendent and staff, setting the expectations for government employees and representing a nineteenth-century sensibility of paternalistic, Protestant-inflected oversight of the less fortunate. "Attendants and nurses are the guardians

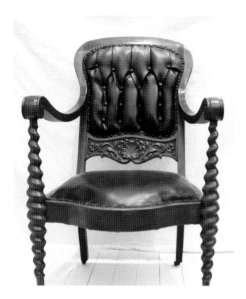
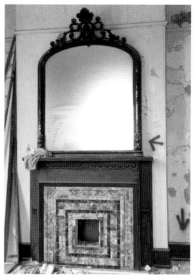

Left: This chair, with spiral turned legs and serpentine front seat rail, was used by medical experts and city leaders in the Center Building's formal boardroom. *Armchair, Center Building, circa 1900, Smithsonian Institution Castle Collection. NBM staff photograph, 2018.*

Right: An ornate fireplace was preserved in a room adjacent to the superintendent's suite. *Photograph, 2015, Caitlin Bristol.*

of the patients, and they must never lose sight of this responsibility…it demands great self control and the exhibition of unusual forbearance and Christian charity."[36]

Even so, constant controversy plagued the hospital administration. As early as 1869—and continually over succeeding decades—newspaper reports charged the head of the hospital with medical neglect of the patients, as well as with failing to provide sufficient food, heat and pay for employees. Charles Nichols, the first superintendent, endured intense scrutiny from Congress, including two thorough investigations. He was called before the secretary of the interior in 1875 to defend the release of certain patients and presented a chart explaining each release. Accusations continued to be leveled at the leadership of the hospital for the next century. A report presented to Congress in 1907 charged Superintendent White with misconduct, alleging abuses by staff as well as insufficient food for patients. In fact, almost every superintendent was criticized for ineffective supervision, treatment, violence and abuse by attendants, insufficient food and unacceptable conditions at the hospital. Although most lawsuits ended

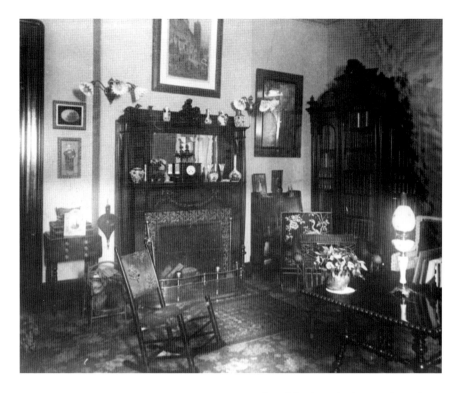

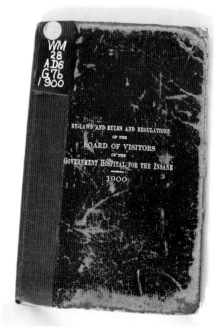

Above: The décor in the superintendent's quarters contributed to a feeling of prestige befitting the leader of a federal hospital. *Photograph, late nineteenth century, U.S. National Library of Medicine.*

Left: The board of visitors outlined the rules and regulations for the superintendent and employees. *From* By-Laws and Rules and Regulations of the Board of Visitors of the Government Hospital for the Insane, *Washington, D.C, 1900, U.S. National Library of Medicine. NBM staff photograph, 2018.*

No.	Name.	Color.	Date of admission.	At whose request.	Place of residence.	Character of case.
1	Reed, Stephen .... *Taken to Prince George's County, Md., June 28, 1875, by District commissioners.	Colored .	7, 29, 1870	Mayor of Washington, D. C.	Not known; supposed to be from Maryland. No relatives or friends known.	Chronic dementia. Not considered violent, but is rather suspicious and sullen. *June, 1875.—No change. Works regularly in stable.
2	Wise, Amelia. .... *August 11, 1875. Remains in the hospital without material change.	White ..	8, 15, 1870	Mayor of Washington, D. C.	Not positively known ; says she lived in Washington and was a midwife. Margaret Hook, living with J. H. Collins, 448 K street northwest, knew something of her.	Chronic dementia. Native of Germany. Generally quiet and dull, but at times violent. *June 30, 1875.—Remains in hospital without material change.
3	Hyne, Charles H .... *Sent to New York, June 15, 1875, by District commissioners.	White ..	1, 19, 1871	Mayor of Washington, D. C.	Nativity, New York City. His mother, Mrs. Sarah K. Hyne, resides at present at 164 East One hundred and twenty-sixth street, Harlem, N. Y.	Congenital imbecility. General health good. Mild and harmless. *June, 1875.—No change. Did considerable wood-work.
4	McGinniss, Patrick .... *Sent to Providence, R. I., June 15, 1875, by District commissioners. August 16, 1875.—Recently learned that this man spent a few days in New York City Asylum on Ward's Island, and then went on his way to Providence.	White ..	4, 24, 1871	Mayor of Washington, D. C.	Not known. He says himself that he has a brother living in Providence, R. I., but have never heard from him.	Chronic mania. Has exalted and extravagant delusions in regard to his own importance, wealth, and position. Not considered violent. About 55 years of age. Has been paralyzed on one side. *June, 1875.—No change.
5	Fitts, Lucy A .... *Sent to Massachusetts by District commissioners, July 2, 1875.—Entirely harmless, and believed to be well able to travel to her home if provided with the means. August 16, 1875.—Recently learned that Miss Fitts reached her home in safety, and has since been placed in the Massachusetts State Lunatic Hospital at Taunton.	White ..	6, 10, 1871	Governor of District of Columbia.	Fitchburgh, Mass. Her father, Robert Fitts, and brothers Robert and Samuel there. A sister, Mrs. T. C. Kenyon, lives in Akron, Ohio.	Chronic dementia. Came to Washington to marry the late Charles Sumner. Will not believe that he is dead, and still determined to marry him. A woman of good education and probably of worthy life.
6	Smith, Woolford .... *Sent to Fredericksburg, Va., June 30, 1875, by District commissioners.	Colored.	8, 26, 1871	Governor of the District of Columbia.	Near Fredericksburgh, Va	Chronic dementia, with epilepsy. Considered a dangerous man. *June, 1875.—Became mild unless molested in the irritable condition that followed a fit.
7	Ten Eyck, Sophronia, alias Henderson.	White ..	2, 16, 1872	Governor of the District of Columbia.	Not known. Says Henry J, Daggett, coal-yard, Cincinnati, Ohio, is her brother-	Chronic mania. No history except what she gives herself. Says a former husband, Ten

14

					Says her maiden name was Sophronia Rand. *Sent to Cincinnati, Ohio, June 15, 1875, by the commissioners of the District of Columbia ; once a patient in Longview Asylum, Hamilton County, Ohio.	in-law, and that John Duboice, well known in Methodist circles in Cincinnati, is her uncle. Have written both parties, and letters returned through dead-letter office.	Eyck, kept a hotel in the city. Is a woman of violent temper and exceedingly abusive with her tongue. Thinks she is maliciously pursued by a man of the name of J. B. Macy. Hears false voices. *June, 1875.—Less under influence of her delusions than formerly, and more manageable, but subject to occasional outbursts of violent language. Is as able, probably, to take care of herself as she had been for a number of years before her admission to the hospital, when she supported herself by selling hair-oil, tracts, &c.
8	Jones, Richard F .... *Taken to Prince George's County, Md., June 28, 1875.	White ..	6, 13, 1872	Governor of the District of Columbia.	Marlborough, Prince George's County, Md. Sister, Mrs. Sarah L. Martin, Uniontown, D. C.	Chronic mania, with delusions. Considered a dangerous man. *June, 1875.—Active manifestations of insanity ceased for several months, and been safely trusted and mild.
9	Barnes, Winneyfurt .... *August 15, 1875.—Remains in hospital.	White ..	6, 20, 1872	Governor of the District of Columbia.	Became insane in Connecticut. Thomas Barnes, her father, lives on Virginia avenue, between First and Second streets, southeast.	Chronic dementia. A tearing, noisy, restless, and sometimes quarrelsome patient. Went to Connecticut three years before admission, and was taken insane there. Said to have been in an asylum in New York City, and then sent home to her father. Age about 24. *June 30, 1875. Not quite as noisy as formerly.
10	Stewart, Eliza H .... *Taken to Prince George's County, Md., June 28, 1875, by District commissioners.	Colored.	9, 9, 1872	Governor of the District of Columbia.	Says she belongs near Marlborough, Prince George's County, Md. No relatives known, but patient says she has brothers living in the city, whose names are Robert, Henry, William, and Charles Stewart.	Chronic dementia. Age about 35. Was picked up in Washington by the police. Noisy, but harmless. *June, 1875.—No material change.
11	Wright, William .... *Sent to Albany, N. Y., June 30, 1875, by District commissioners.	White ..	10, 3, 1872	Governor of the District of Columbia.	Not known. He says himself that he has a brother living at Albany, N. Y.	Chronic mania. Quiet and manageable under proper supervision, but an unsafe person to be at large. *June, 1875.—After above report was prepared, we learned that this man had been in prison at Auburn, N. Y., for theft, and transferred to Asylum for Criminal Lunatics, and discharged therefrom as fit to be at large.
12	Witzell, James............. *Sent to West Virginia, June 15, 1875, by District commissioners.	White ..	10, 7, 1872	Governor of the District of Columbia.	His supposed residence is somewhere in Western Virginia; the address of friends and relatives not known.	A harmless imbecile. *June, 1875.—No change.
13	Campbell, Bridget .... *Taken to New York, July 2, 1875, by District commissioners.	White ..	12, 12, 1872	Governor of the District of Columbia.	Not known. Says she has been a type-setter in New York City, and has been in the asylum at Utica, N. Y.	Chronic dementia. Native of Ireland. Age about 40. Patient is generally very quiet, but sometimes violent. Nothing known of her except what she tells herself. *June, 1875.—Became more demented and passive, and rarely violent.

15

Superintendent Nichols was called before the secretary of the interior in 1875 to defend the release of certain patients. *From* Report and Correspondence Relating to the Release from the Government Hospital for the Insane, *U.S. Government Printing Office, 1875, Library Collection, Historical Society of Washington, D.C.*

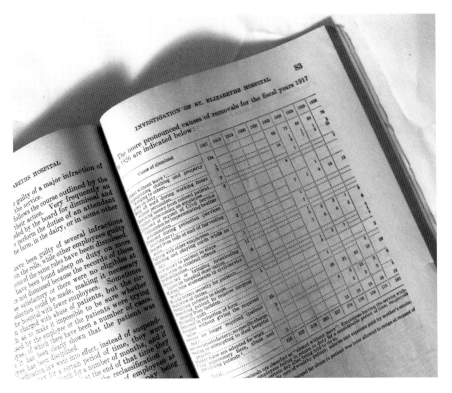

Congressional investigations charged the head of the hospital with medical neglect of the patients, as well as providing insufficient food, heat and pay for employees. *From* Investigation of St. Elizabeths Hospital, *U.S. General Accounting Office, 1926, U.S. National Library of Medicine. NBM staff photograph, 2018.*

without penalty, the hospital temporarily lost accreditation in the 1970s, while still under federal control, and then in the 1980s after its transfer to the District of Columbia. Even in recent years, accusations against hospital administrators continue to make headlines.

While the superintendents remained under scrutiny, a large staff helped manage the large residential hospital with many moving parts. As at other large institutions founded in the nineteenth century, including private schools and military bases, many employees of St. Elizabeths lived on campus. Staff members, who, other than the nurses and some female attendants, were usually hired as single men, might marry during their tenure at the hospital and live with their families.

At first, it was easier to house staff on campus. In many of the areas— such as the bakery, laundry, cemetery and fire station—the staff members

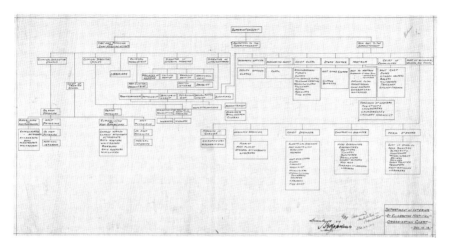

The staff at the hospital continued to grow with the patient population. *Document, 1919, Library of Congress, American Architectural Foundation Collection.*

lived in proximity to their work. Single staff members found space in residential buildings or wherever there was extra room. In the 1860s, about 110 people worked at St. Elizabeths, including attendants, doctors, housekeepers, cooks, a horticulturist, a kitchen steward, farmers, maids, engineers and carpenters. As part of Superintendent Richardson's modernization plan for the campus after 1900, service functions were moved and consolidated, increasing efficiency. The addition of a new storehouse allowed for the modernization and standardization of distributing goods around campus, leading to less waste. New buildings also provided housing for workers so that they could move out of the patient wards.

Superintendent White oversaw construction of seven staff residences in the 1920s, to be occupied by the heads of the departments and physicians who lived on campus with their families. Some of these wood-frame structures were two-story, vernacular houses in the four-square style. Toward the end of the twentieth century, as the tradition of on-campus living waned, attendants, laborers, researchers and other staff migrated to surrounding neighborhoods such as Anacostia and Congress Heights, establishing strong and long-lasting hospital/community ties and sometimes even multigenerational families of employees.

By the 1930s, the hospital employed a staff of 1,600, and by the end of World War II, staff numbered almost 4,000. By this time, self-sufficiency was rendered impractical, and most of the staff no longer lived on campus.

As the hospital organization and administration modernized in the early twentieth century, paternalistic practices and the village life of the hospital began to fade. The government began collecting payment for room and board from staff beginning in the 1930s. The hospital grounds began to resemble a twentieth-century government facility rather than a self-sufficient, isolated town.

RECREATION

Most wards had jump ropes, badminton sets, checkers (regular and Chinese), bingo, bean bags, scrabble, dominoes, jigsaw puzzles, ring toss, coloring books, croquet sets, horse shoes, record players, and ping pong equipment.[37]
—St. Elizabeths Hospital Memorandum, 1956

St. Elizabeths' patients and staff participated in a wide range of cultural, educational and entertainment activities. In the 1880s, there was even briefly a small zoo—including caged bear cubs—on the campus for the enjoyment of the patients. A permanent venue, Hitchcock Hall, was built in 1908 as an arts and recreation hub for patients and staff and named after Secretary of the Interior Ethan A. Hitchcock. With its terra-cotta embellishment, Hitchcock Hall is one of the most architecturally sophisticated structures on campus. The building's 1,200-seat auditorium hosted meeting space for assemblies, as well as cultural activities such as movies, operas, musicals, dances and lectures, giving institutionalized patients a glimpse of the outside world. The employee orchestra played there; volunteers from the Department of the Interior presented slideshows of National Park images; and patients, usually in segregated audiences, could see performances by, for example, the acrobatic Del Ray Brothers, John Philip Sousa and the U.S. Marine Band.

Starting in 1919, the American Red Cross set up an office at St. Elizabeths to provide a racially segregated entertainment program for veterans that included baseball games, dances and brief excursions into the city. The organization constructed a building next to Hitchcock Hall and provided services that included working with veterans to help them build skills for life outside the hospital. The Red Cross also held athletic competitions and field days. The Knights of Columbus also set up a shop on campus in the 1920s, where the group oversaw classes in woodworking, toy making and other crafts, also restricted to veterans.

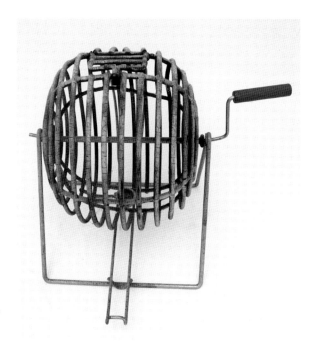

Recreational activities on the patient wards included bingo. *Bingo sorter, found in the Center Building, U.S. General Services Administration. NBM staff photograph, 2018.*

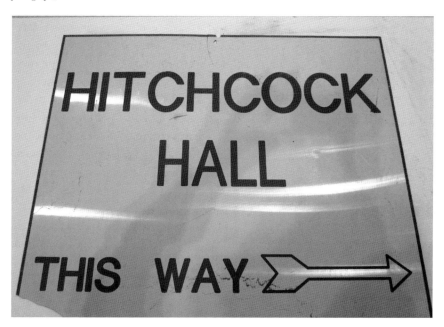

Hitchcock Hall's 1,200-seat auditorium hosted meeting space for assemblies as well as cultural activities for patients such as movies, operas, musicals, dances and lectures. *Sign, twentieth century, U.S. General Services Administration. NBM staff photograph, 2018.*

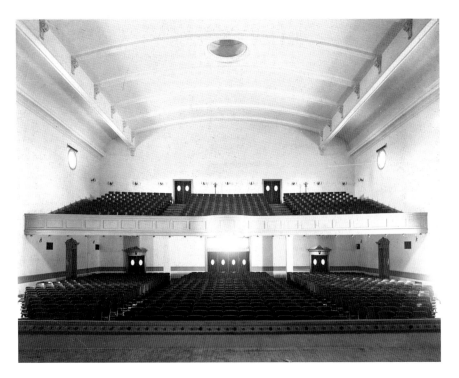

Hitchcock Hall was opened in 1908 as a theater for assemblies, performances and entertainment on campus. *Photograph, circa 1910, National Archives and Records Administration (418-G-141).*

Superintendents encouraged the hospital staff and patients to participate in various forms of recreation together—although sometimes these activities went awry. In 1906, an investigation accused the staff of gambling with their charges, noting that "cards were played for money by the attendants and patients."[38] Staff did work with patients to form musical bands, although the administration did not always speak positively about the musical program at the hospital. Superintendent Godding once noted that although there were some talented military musicians among the patients, it often sounded as though "evil spirits get into their horns."[39]

In general, patients, segregated by race and gender, participated in some familiar activities from outside life. Over the years, many patients participated in sports, including baseball, boxing, croquet and golf. Teams of male patients and staff played baseball off and on over the years as part of the Washington, D.C., amateur league. African American men at Howard Hall, perhaps not allowed on the baseball field, were offered

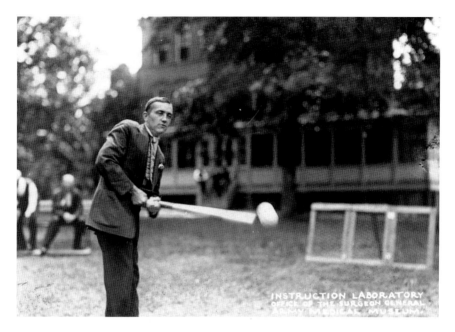

Teams of patients and staff played baseball off and on over the years, with the hospital's team playing in the Washington, D.C., amateur league. *Photograph, early twentieth century, National Museum of Health and Medicine.*

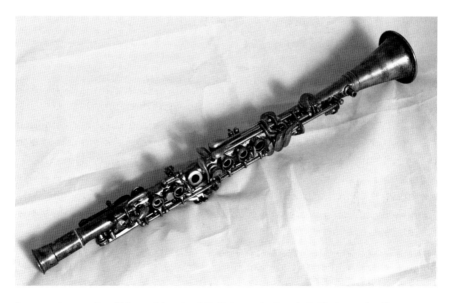

Some patients and staff formed bands while living at the hospital. *Clarinet used at St. Elizabeths, twentieth century, National Museum of Health and Medicine. NBM staff photograph, 2018.*

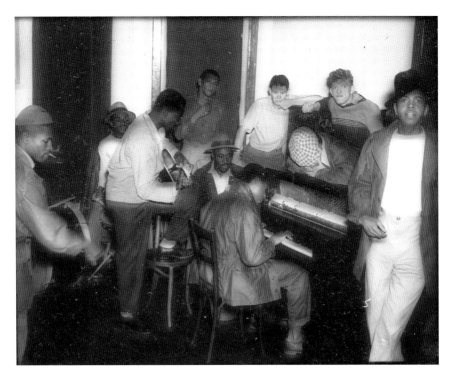

Patients around the piano. *Photograph, early twentieth century, National Museum of Health and Medicine.*

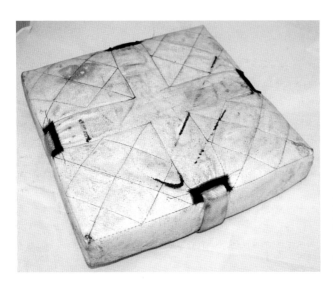

Bases used at St. Elizabeths, from the twentieth century. *U.S. General Services Administration. NBM staff photograph, 2018.*

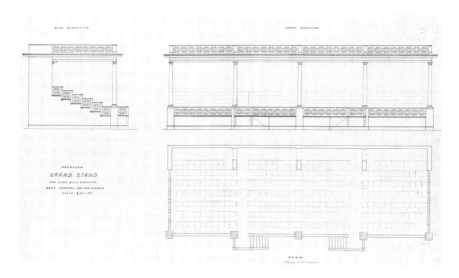

This grandstand, though never built, indicates that leaders at the hospital wanted to be able to host large events outside, whether baseball games or other assemblies. *Drawing, circa 1910, Library of Congress, American Architectural Foundation Collection.*

facilities for boxing. In 1927, a women's beauty shop, staffed by nurses who had beauty school training or experience, was established in the Toner Building, the white women's infirmary. Superintendent William White explained his motivation in funding such an endeavor: "The beauty treatment gives our women patients self-respect. It bucks them up, makes them take an interest in life."[40]

Reading was also an important pastime at the hospital. The circulating library was first housed in the Center Building, where, in 1912, librarian Louise Sackman Hough catalogued the library books. Books arrived at the hospital from many sources, including directly to veterans through the Soldiers and Sailors Camp Library, a program that delivered almost 10 million books to service members during World War I. The inventory included many histories, biographies and novels, such as classic volumes by Louisa May Alcott, Nathaniel Hawthorne, George Eliot and Charles Dickens. Outgrowing the space and needing to be more accessible to patients around campus, the library moved into the former mortuary and laboratory, the Rest Building, in 1929, with bookshelves and reading rooms on the first floor.

Not much is known about the daily life of resident youth and how it may have differed significantly from that for adults at the hospital. Over

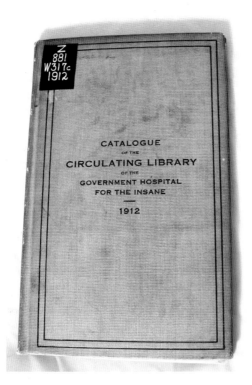

Left: The library inventory included many histories, biographies and novels, such as volumes by Louisa May Alcott, Nathaniel Hawthorne, George Eliot and Charles Dickens. *Catalogue of the Circulating Library of the Government Hospital for the Insane, Book, 1912, U.S. National Library of Medicine. NBM staff photograph, 2018.*

Below: Patients had access to a circulating library, with bookshelves and reading rooms on the first floor of the old mortuary building. *Photograph, mid-twentieth century, U.S. National Library of Medicine.*

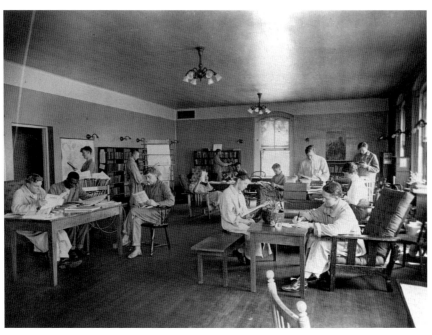

the course of the hospital's history, there were likely always some teenagers in care. In 1869, for example, Superintendent Nichols admitted the fifteen-year-old daughter of a Maryland lighthouse keeper, and in 1937, a fifteen-year-old patient made the news after she was accused of killing an older patient while in hospital custody. Older teenagers always made up some part of the patient population, although their numbers were relatively small. Targeted youth programs did not exist until 1962, at which time there were more than fifty young people in residence, five of whom were under twelve years old. In 1964, a new Youth Center separated children from adults and offered special services.

Patients came to St. Elizabeths from all religious backgrounds, although mandatory chapel attendance was once part of the treatment program. Most patients were Protestant or Catholic, but hospital staff provided opportunities for those of other faiths to worship during their stay on campus. Local clergy often came to assist in religious rituals, such as leading a Passover Seder for Jewish residents. Chapel space had long been provided in the Center Building and elsewhere on campus in lieu of a special building for that purpose. The Center Building's third-floor auditorium hosted short religious assemblies as well as other secular activities. Longtime chaplain Ernie Bruder fought for a designated building for religious services on campus. "It is a scandal to the hospital," he wrote in 1948, "that a small, inadequate room, never designated for the purpose, and used for any and all other purposes, should have to serve as the hospital Chapel."[41] A new, purpose-built chapel was constructed on the East Campus in 1955 in the Colonial Revival style with a prominent brick bell tower. Its interior stained-glass windows honored the service of Chaplain Bruder to the hospital community.

MEDICAL CARE AND TREATMENT

The doctrine of moral treatment slowly gave way to a more scientific methodology for patient care at the turn of the twentieth century. Although the ideas of empathy, fresh air and productive work were hardly formally rebuked, new understandings about neuropsychology changed the best practices of hospital care for the mentally ill. Over time, St. Elizabeths' doctors, attendants and nurses tried all sorts of treatments and cures—both common and innovative—including dance, art therapy, psychodrama, animal therapy, drugs and physical restraints. Race, gender and sexual orientation prejudices on the part of the staff, as well as overcrowding and understaffing in general, informed the treatment plans. All the doctors developing the protocols for the hospital, and most of those administering the various treatments, were white men for its first half century and beyond. St. Elizabeths hired its first permanent female doctor, Mary O'Malley, for the women's wards in 1905, and it became the first public mental health hospital in the nation to train medical interns in the 1920s.

At the turn of the twentieth century, Superintendent Richardson enacted new procedures mandating more complete medical history reporting and other scientific approaches to patient care. Although science was taking center stage at American asylums, with new technologies and treatment regimens, old methods often persisted in new guises. Hydrotherapy for mental illness, for example, is an ancient technique. George Foster introduced the practice at St. Elizabeths, first in the Toner and Oak wards for white men and subsequently for white women. African American patients had access to hydrotherapy only after buildings were renovated in later decades. Hydrotherapy used specially designed baths to submerge

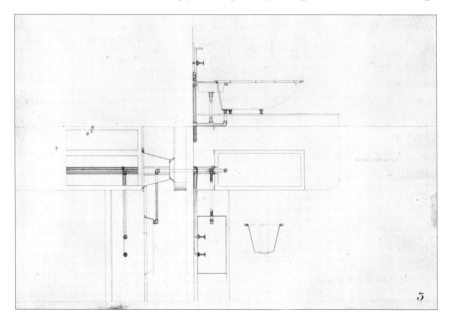

Used to shock or calm patients, specially designed baths were installed in 1897 for use on white men. *Drawing, circa 1890s, Library of Congress, American Architectural Foundation Collection.*

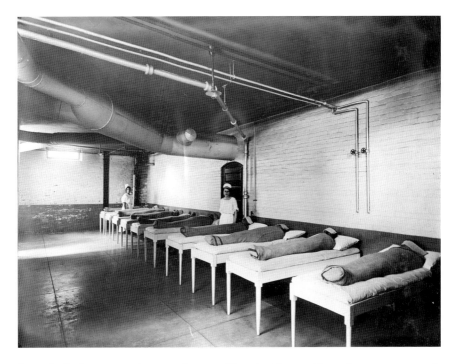

In one hydrotherapy practice, attendants would wet bedsheets with varying temperatures of water, wrap the patients and wait for several hours. *Photograph, circa 1900, National Archives and Records Administration (418-P-634).*

patients in either hot or cold water for several hours to either shock or calm them. In one hydrotherapy practice, attendants would wet bedsheets with varying temperatures of water, wrap the patients and wait for the treatment to take effect. Hot water was used for patients with insomnia, while cold water was used on manic patients. By the 1920s, thousands of patients were receiving hydrotherapy.

The use of electroshock therapy reached its apex in the 1950s. Now known as electroconvulsive therapy, the procedure is still used in certain cases. Electroshock therapy induces a seizure with the goal of altering brain chemistry to improve the patient's mental state. Today, this type of treatment is an option reserved for those with severe depression and is only administered when the patient is under anesthesia.

The teachings of psychotherapist Sigmund Freud peaked in influence in midcentury. Diagnoses of mental illness and understanding of disease often relied heavily on an understanding of family influence. At St. Elizabeths, as at other asylums, many practitioners focused on invented

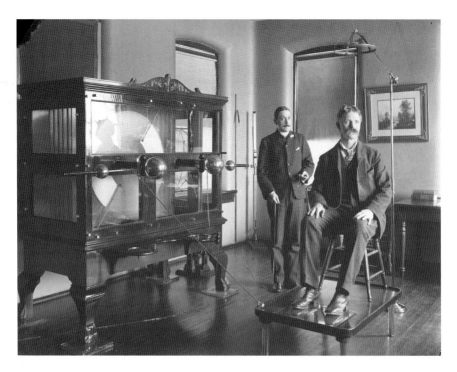

An "old electric shock machine" was used in the Toner Building at St. Elizabeths in the early twentieth century. *Photograph, circa 1920s, National Archives and Records Administration (418-G-313).*

definitions of sexual depravity to explain mental illness. As part of the diagnosis of patient "JF," for example, St. Elizabeths' staff noted that the patient had "quarrelsome parents" and was "too closely associated with the mother," suggesting that the mental illness was caused by the family itself. Complex charts from the hospital dating from the 1950s illustrate a medical emphasis on the patient's family history, sexuality and alcohol usage. In one case, the doctor noted "bad" hereditary as well as environmental influences and both repressed "homosexual tendencies" and "heterosexual maladjustment." Many patients arrived with histories of sexual assault or incest. Others were labeled as homosexuals, which was then considered grounds for a diagnosis of mental instability and even psychosis. Gay patients, whose sexuality made up the mental illness diagnosis, received some of the same treatments as other patients, including electric shock and hydrotherapy.

Lobotomy, a surgical operation to remove part of the brain, was once considered to be a genuine way to subdue and cure patients. Dr. Walter

Freeman, a practicing psychiatrist at St. Elizabeths hospital, did not believe that the "talk cure," or psychotherapy, would work for most patients and searched for a surgical cure instead. He performed his first lobotomy in 1936. After altering his procedure over time—even developing a method to access the brain through the eye socket—Freeman would eventually perform 2,500 lobotomies on patients in twenty-three states. Fewer than 100 of these took place at St. Elizabeths, as Superintendent Overholser and other staff members discouraged the practice. Eventually, about 20,000 people underwent the procedure nationwide. Lobotomy subdued the patient and made him or her more docile and "child-like" and, therefore, easier to monitor and control from the perspective of hospital staff. In many cases, the patient never regained his or her full control or abilities. Even from the beginning, lobotomy was widely criticized within the field. Informed consent did not exist, and families were not always aware of the risks. Lobotomy was often performed on the poorest patients, as in the 1952 West Virginia Lobotomy Project, in which 238 patients at the Lakin State Hospital for the Colored Insane were lobotomized in one month. With the advent of drugs to treat psychosis in the mid-1950s, the age of lobotomy came to an end. Freeman closed his practice in D.C. and moved to California, where he promoted lobotomy for depressed housewives and as a cure for hyperactivity in children. Freeman performed his last lobotomy, on a patient who died from the procedure, in 1967, after which his medical privileges were revoked.

Medications, including opium and alkaline bromides, were historically employed to subdue the mentally ill. In the nineteenth century, doctors also used hydrate of chloral and other hypnotics to assist in patient care. Beginning in the 1950s with tranquilizing drugs such as Thorazine, and continuing in later decades with Prozac and other therapies, drugs assumed a greater role in helping patients leave the hospital to live on their own.

Despite the (in most cases deserved) reputation for draconian measures at mental health hospitals nationwide, there were examples of care that were beneficial and noninvasive. Art therapy, according to lithographer Prentiss Taylor, could "help a patient to maintain, or make momentarily better, or reestablish what he can of his world."[42] Taylor worked with patients at St. Elizabeths from 1943 to 1954 and hosted exhibitions of their art. His well-received show celebrating patient art premiered at the Federal Security Agency in Washington, D.C., before traveling to other sites. The display received much attention from mental health institutions across the country. He also wrote an influential article about art therapy

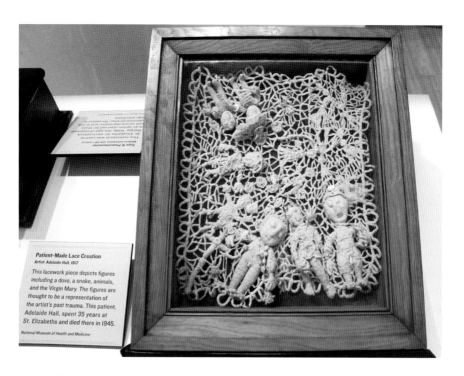

Above: *Patient-made lace creation, artist Adelaide Hall, 1917, National Museum of Health and Medicine. NBM staff photograph, 2018.*

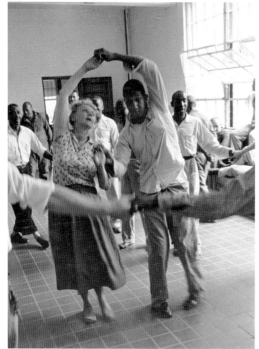

Left: Marian Chace, internationally known as the founder of dance therapy, led the program at St. Elizabeths for several decades. *Photograph, circa 1960s, St. Elizabeths Hospital Museum.*

in 1950 for the *American Journal of Psychiatry*. With his patients, Taylor used watercolors, oils, pencils and charcoal in a therapeutic setting. Often the art reflected complex feelings and perspectives.

For many decades, Marian Chace, credited with founding the field of dance therapy in the United States, led that program at St. Elizabeths. Chace worked with the team of doctors and therapists in patient conferences and other clinical and educational work. Her patients included both acute, short-term residents and chronic, long-term cases. Holding the dance therapy sessions on the wards allowed patients to come and go as they felt comfortable. Over her tenure at St. Elizabeths, Chace and her patients performed pieces for staff and visitors, showcasing her work as well as providing patients a way to communicate to others about what life was like in a hospital through dance. For the Centennial of the hospital in 1955, celebrated in grand fashion with local dignitaries and medical personnel, the dancers performed "We the Mentally Ill," an original dance highlighting the history of Dorothea Dix's role in founding the hospital in 1855 after visiting the mentally ill in jails across New England.

In 1941, St. Elizabeths patients participated in a new kind of treatment: psychodrama. Originally developed by J.L. Moreno of Ohio's Beacon Hill Sanitarium, psychodramatic therapy encouraged participants to act out events from their past or to practice behaving appropriately in everyday encounters. Sessions took place in Hitchcock Hall. Patients used psychodramatic therapy to gain confidence and skills before returning to the unpredictable world beyond the hospital's walls. A May 1941 report in the medical journal *Sociometry* described the case of a young man at St. Elizabeths who overcame social anxiety by attending psychodrama sessions, first as an audience member and later as a performer.

In the nineteenth century, attendants administered generalized day-to-day care rather than nurses. Like other segments of the workforce looking to improve job conditions, St. Elizabeths' attendants joined the Hospital Attendants' Protective Union in 1900. They used their labor collectively to agitate for better pay and working conditions soon after, when they leveled various complaints against management under the new superintendent, William White, in 1904.

A nursing school operated on site from 1894 to 1952, and this new population of trained nurses took over many of the tasks that had been performed by attendants. Nursing students lived on campus and received hands-on education in both medical supervision and day-to-day patient care. The duties of a nurse at St. Elizabeths were often difficult. In fact, a hospital publication in 1900 called the job "most trying," noting that the position would "require the highest type of character."[43] In 1908, Superintendent White expanded the reach of the nursing school, noting that only half of the wards had nurses overseeing patients. The remaining wards were under the watch of attendants with no medical training. In 1923, a preliminary training course for nurses at St. Elizabeths provided detailed instructions on making beds, scrubbing equipment, admitting patients and other tasks.

The site's first home for nurses, the E Building, was part of the Shepley, Rutan & Coolidge–designed expansion. The new building exemplified the increasing professionalization of the hospital's medical staff in the early twentieth century. A handbook laying out strict rules welcomed nurses to their residence at Barton Hall, constructed on the East Campus in 1945.

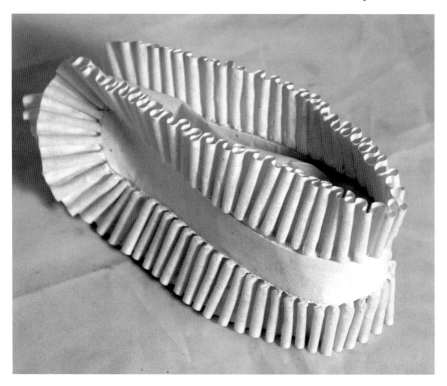

Nurses helped provide professional care to patients in all aspects of their daily lives. *Hat, early twentieth century, National Museum of Health and Medicine, donated by a nurse at St. Elizabeths who trained at the Philadelphia General Hospital. NBM staff photograph, 2018.*

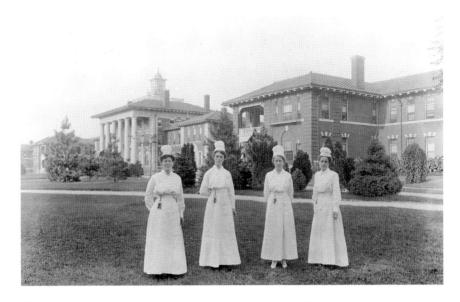

Nursing students lived on campus and received hands-on training in both medical supervision and day-to-day patient care. *Photograph, circa 1920s, National Archives and Records Administration (418-P-644).*

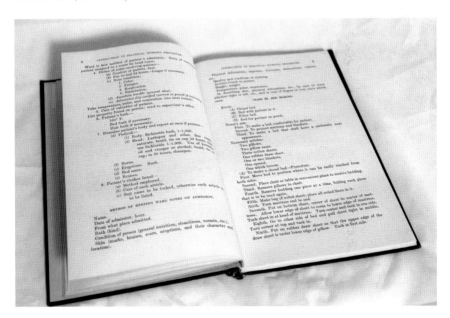

This preliminary training course for nurses at St. Elizabeths provided detailed instructions on making beds, scrubbing equipment, admitting patients and other tasks. *From* Course of Instruction in Practical Nursing as Given in the Training School for Nurses at St. Elizabeths Hospital, *Government Printing Office, 1923, U.S. National Library of Medicine. NBM staff photograph, 2018.*

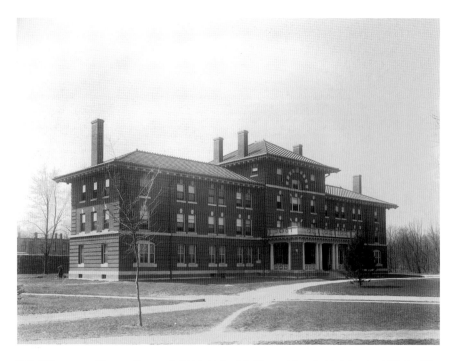

E Building, nurses' home. *Photograph, 1910, National Archives and Records Administration (418-G-115).*

Nurses had to follow procedures for everything from curfews and proper bed-making to playing music. The instructions noted, for example, that smoking should not be done "indiscriminately on the grounds."

RESEARCH

In 1884, Superintendent Godding established a pathology laboratory at St. Elizabeths, the first at any mental health institution in the United States. He believed that funding brain research would lead to the next insights and treatments for mental illness. The Rest Building, built in 1882, housed the original mortuary and pathology laboratory at St. Elizabeths. In a report to Congress in 1905, administrators noted, "[W]e have located here a revolving autopsy table and an arc light, so that work can be done readily at night."[44] The Rest Building reflects a change in thinking about

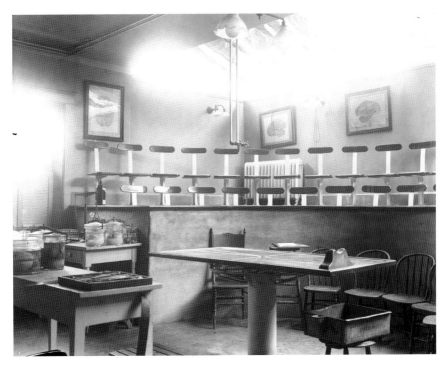

The Rest Building, built in 1882, was the original mortuary and pathology laboratory at St. Elizabeths. *Photograph, 1915, National Archives and Records Administration (418-G-288).*

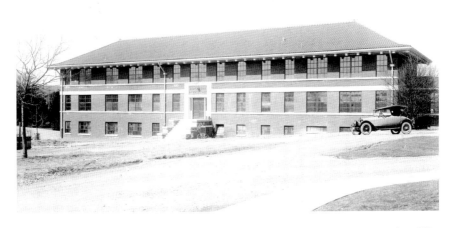

Operational until 2010, Blackburn Laboratory was the longest-running laboratory in a U.S. mental institution. *Photograph, 1925, National Archives and Records Administration (418-G-58).*

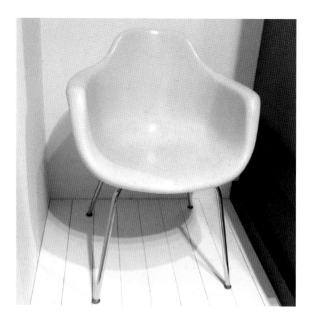

Chairs from the Blackburn Laboratory's autopsy gallery are now used for visitors at the new hospital. *Autopsy theater chair, mid-twentieth century, St. Elizabeths Hospital Museum. NBM staff photograph, 2018.*

mental illness. Using autopsy and the new study of psychopathology, scientists began to learn more about brain function and organ function as they sought a long-term understanding of mental illness.

St. Elizabeths had one of the country's first psychology laboratories, and in 1910, Superintendent White created a new research-focused department including psychologists, pathologists and technicians. Due to the hospital's top reputation, as well as its superintendents' prominent role in the national field of psychiatry, many of the twentieth century's leading practitioners worked at or visited St. Elizabeths. For example, Carl Jung, a proponent of psychoanalysis, arrived in 1912 to study the dreams of African American patients. In the mid-twentieth century, National Institute of Mental Health researchers administered tests to patients at St. Elizabeths to measure memory and verbal and nonverbal skills to better develop treatment plans.

Built in 1923 and operational until 2010, Blackburn Laboratory was the longest-running laboratory in a U.S. mental institution. Built in the Italian Renaissance Revival style that dominates the architecture of the East Campus, the laboratory was nonetheless modern in the interior design of the autopsy gallery in the basement level. The molded fiberglass chairs for invited observers, copies of a classic midcentury modern design, complemented the state-of-the-art scientific proceedings. Using autopsy and the new study of psychopathology, scientists began to learn more about the possible physical manifestations of mental illness.

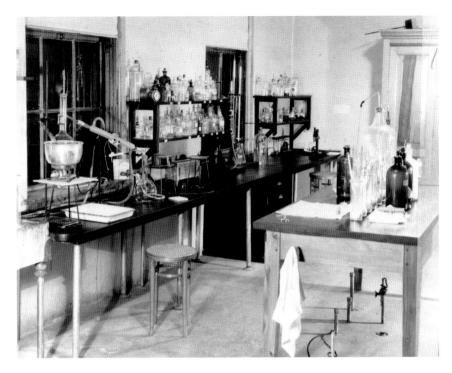

In 1884, Superintendent Godding established a pathology laboratory, the first such at an institution in the United States, out of a belief that funding brain research would lead to the next insights and treatments for mental illness. *Photograph, 1910, U.S. National Library of Medicine.*

Using the extensive bank of brain tissue collected at the laboratory, researchers studied degenerative brain disorders, making important discoveries. *Brain tissue glass plates, mid-twentieth century, St. Elizabeths Hospital Museum. NBM staff photograph, 2018.*

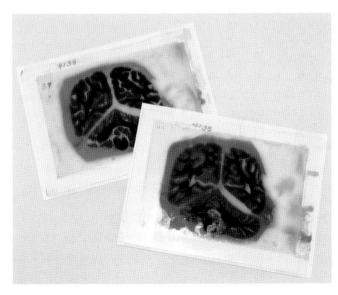

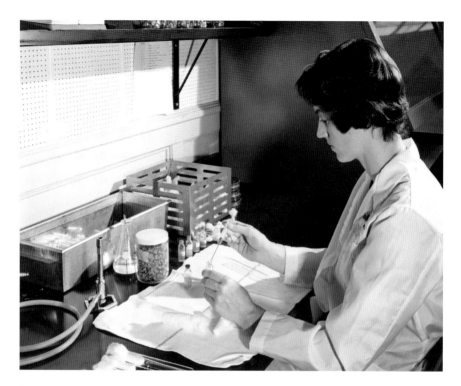

Using autopsy and the new study of psychopathology, scientists began to learn more about the possible physical manifestations of mental illness. *Photograph, mid-twentieth century, U.S. National Library of Medicine.*

The laboratory was named after Isaac Wright Blackburn, a pathologist and scientific director who had worked at the hospital from 1884 to 1911. Blackburn, a talented medical artist, produced *Illustrations of the Gross Morbid Anatomy of the Brain in the Insane.* The 1908 tome featured seventy-five plates illustrating—in many cases for the first time—different pathological conditions of the brain, including acute dementia, alongside descriptions of patient symptoms and family histories. Meta Neumann, a neuropathologist at St. Elizabeths for almost fifty years, also used the laboratory's extensive bank of brain tissue to study degenerative brain disorders. She made important discoveries on conditions such as Alzheimer's disease.

The prolific research done at the Blackburn Laboratory was a gift to the future: a long-term study of brain diseases could not help contemporary patients but furthered later breakthroughs. The Blackburn-Neumann Collection of brain tissue resides now at the National Museum of Health and

Medicine and is a resource for neuromedical researchers. While the laboratory is now closed, the collection of detailed case histories, glass slides with brain specimens and five thousand photographs from fifteen thousand autopsies of St. Elizabeths patients continues to aid researchers.

PART V
THE END OF AN ERA

DEINSTITUTIONALIZATION

Many such hospitals and homes have been shamefully understaffed, overcrowded, unpleasant institutions.... The time has come for a bold new approach.[45]
—John F. Kennedy, 1963

In 1963, President John F. Kennedy made a major announcement about the future of the federal government's role in mental health care: "We must move from the outmoded use of distant custodial institutions to the concept of community-centered agencies."[46] He envisioned a network—never realized—of 1,500 small community mental health clinics across the country that could replace crowded, deteriorating, underfunded public hospitals.

Nationwide, deinstitutionalization began in the 1960s and continued for several decades as the federal and state governments disinvested from their own mental health care infrastructure. The Social Security Amendment Act of 1965, which created Medicaid and Medicare, specifically prohibited Medicare from providing coverage for adults who received long-term care in mental health institutions. Funding and staffing for community clinics fell behind, and by the mid-1970s the population of psychiatric hospitals in the United States was less than half of its 1955 peak. Further cutbacks in federal spending for mental health care came in the 1980s. President Jimmy Carter's Mental Health Systems Act of 1980, which would have provided federal funding to

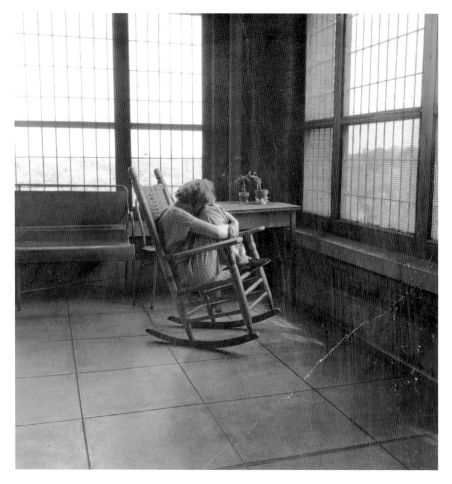

St. Elizabeths patient in a rocking chair. *Photograph, 1955, U.S. National Library of Medicine.*

clinics, was quickly overturned by President Ronald Reagan's administration with the Omnibus Budget Bill of 1981. This bill sharply reduced federal funding for mental health care by substituting direct funding with block grants to the states. However, at the state level, legislatures also limited funding for public clinics and hospitals, and the money tended to be reallocated. By 1990, the nationwide population at mental health hospitals had fallen still further, to around one-fifth of the peak in 1955. At St. Elizabeths, the population dropped from 8,000 to 1,500 in three decades.

By the late twentieth century, many large hospitals had closed for good, having shed tens of thousands of patients. Inpatient care decreased due to many factors beyond the loss of federal and state funding. These included the development and increased use of antipsychotic drugs and a new movement championing the rights and independence of the mentally ill. Patient-rights activists hoped that outpatients, whom they called consumers of care, would be better able to live on their own, although this was not always the case. By the early 1980s, in part due to patients leaving public hospitals, up to one-third of America's growing homeless population was affected by schizophrenia, schizoaffective disorder, bipolar disorder or major depression. Residential hospitals no longer existed to care for them.

The architecture of mental health care shifted from large campuses of custodial care to a combination of small outpatient clinics, nursing homes, chronic illness hospitals, foster homes and halfway houses. The age of the asylum was over.

KIRKBRIDES ACROSS AMERICA

Out of the almost eighty Kirkbride hospitals that once served patients across America, about thirty-five are still standing in some form today, including the Center Building on the St. Elizabeths West Campus. Some remain on the grounds of psychiatric hospitals, a handful of which remain in active use. Some have been repurposed for other uses, such as condominiums or nursing homes. The majority stand vacant, awaiting adaptive use or facing neglect and eventual demolition. Across the nation, Kirkbride buildings have a complex historical legacy and will continue to present a challenge for historic preservationists.

The public's understanding of mental health and mental health hospitals has always been complex and makes garnering needed support for preserving and rehabilitating these old structures challenging in some markets. Often these hospitals have been major employers in a region and have provided important help in difficult times. However, memory is long, and some families resent the overcrowding and inferior care they felt their loved ones received in these institutions. Public perceptions of desolate corridors and despairing patients make reuse of buildings associated with the mentally ill challenging.

Over the centuries, relentless negative publicity and periodic exposés of mental health care facilities have consumed the popular culture. As early as the late nineteenth century, writers have reported sordid stories about life

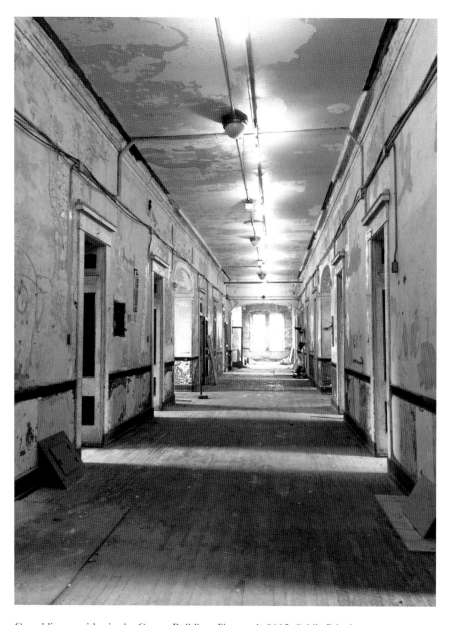

Crumbling corridor in the Center Building. *Photograph, 2015, Caitlin Bristol.*

inside the walls of an asylum. Nelly Bly's *Ten Days in a Madhouse* (1887) was a lurid tale in which the reporter went undercover at the women's lunatic asylum on Blackwell Island in New York City. Clifford Beers's *A Mind that Found Itself* (1908) is credited with ushering in the modern patients-rights movement. The late twentieth-century classic film *One Flew Over the Cuckoo's Nest* (1975), based on Ken Kesey's 1962 book, was filmed in a Kirkbride building at the Oregon State Hospital in Salem. These and other dark, upsetting depictions of asylums—*Shutter Island* (2003, with the film version in 2010) is but one twenty-first-century example—encouraged the public to think critically about the future of institutionalization of the mentally ill and helped explain some ambivalence in communities seeking to raise funds to preserve these structures and tell their complicated histories.

Some advocates of historic asylums include urban explorers and paranormal enthusiasts, forming unusual bonds with historic preservationists. Kirkbrides—standing empty on large, desolate campuses and surrounded by unmarked graves—attract people looking for "haunted" history. Urban explorers seize on ruins for unique and picturesque adventure amid melancholy vistas of peeling paint in deserted corridors. Some mental health advocates criticize this interest as macabre and inappropriate. However, ghost hunters and other "place hackers" have emerged as leaders of the movement to preserve these threatened buildings. Instagrammers and other photographers often find beauty in the ruins of old mental health hospitals. Ghost tours, such as those offered by the Trans-Allegheny Lunatic Asylum in West Virginia, promise that "the Asylum has had apparition sightings, unexplainable voices and sounds, and other paranormal activity reported in the past." The museum welcomes visitors to take a late-night tour of its Kirkbride building and "decide for yourself if [patients are] still occupying the historic wards and treatment rooms."[47]

Often, the efforts of historic preservation activists are not enough to save a hospital. The Lunatic Asylum at Morristown, New Jersey, known as Greystone, opened in 1876. A century later, after falling into disuse, the building attracted a following of historic preservationists who tried to prevent its demolition. State officials did not agree that the building was salvageable and demolished the historic structure in 2015. Preservationists hope to erect a permanent memorial on the site using some of its original material.

Despite the losses, developers across the country are discovering new and creative uses for some of these complicated and unwieldy buildings. A number of former psychiatric hospitals have been successfully adapted as condominiums, shops, restaurants and hotels. For example, Kirkbride Hall at what was once

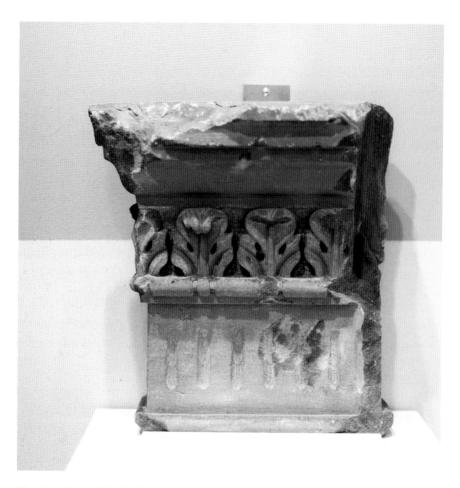

The demolition of Morris Plains, New Jersey's Greystone Asylum was a blow to preservationists. They hope to erect a permanent memorial on the site and repurpose some of the original material. *Architectural fragment from demolition, 2015, courtesy of Robert Duffy. Photo by Yassine El Mansouri, 2017.*

Traverse State Hospital in Michigan has been a popular site for meetings, events and weddings. Its website notes that "the stunning renovated structure and the history of beauty and humanity behind its name have created a truly remarkable and unique place."[48] The hospital grounds—now known as the Village at Grand Traverse Commons—hosts festivals, farmers' markets and guided historic tours. Buffalo, New York, boasts another success story, at the former home of the Buffalo State Hospital for the Insane. The Kirkbride building there was designed by well-known architect H.H. Richardson, and landscape architects Frederick Law Olmsted and Calvert Vaux designed the grounds. After patients moved out in the 1970s, the building fell into disrepair. Following decades of subsequent debate about the future of the empty building, Buffalo's leaders approved a development plan for the aging Kirkbride building with its iconic copper roof. Olmsted and Vaux's expansive lawn, which had been converted to a parking lot, was re-landscaped. After extensive renovation, the complex opened a luxury hotel, the Hotel Henry Urban Resort Conference Center, in 2017. The building shares space with the Buffalo Architecture Center.

Despite the promise of moral treatment, Kirkbride buildings faced challenges that led to overcrowding and criticism. Government-funded budgets fell short of what was needed to maintain staff levels, proper building conditions and patient privacy. Campuses designed to promote healing and hope came, instead, to symbolize the difficult lives many patients led while hospitalized. By the late twentieth century, large underfunded custodial hospitals, no longer equipped to provide a curative environment, had lost much of the public's trust. Complicating the potential for historic preservation even further, most of these structures had been vacant for several decades and require significant resources to properly rehabilitate. Despite such obstacles, many activists strongly believe that Americans need to openly reckon with the complex history of mental health care by preserving the remaining examples of Kirkbride hospitals, and city leaders see the benefits of economic redevelopment.

D.C. TAKES OVER

The tradition of this place is not what we've heard about in the last 20 years. The tradition of this place is the forefront of psychiatry in the world.[49]
—Patrick J. Canavan, 2010

A hospital for the mentally ill has operated continuously on the old St. Elizabeths tract since 1855. When Dorothea Dix and her colleagues recommended best practices for housing people with mental illness in the mid-nineteenth century, they believed that such an institution should house 250 patients, which is about the same number in residence at St. Elizabeths Hospital today. Of course, with the nation's population vastly increased, this represents a far smaller commitment to public mental health care than in previous generations.

By the 1960s, as the age of the large, state-sponsored hospital ended, the federal government began a "planned, phased, gradual transfer of Saint Elizabeths Hospital to the District of Columbia."[50] Overcrowding as well as persistent complaints about patient care and facility maintenance had plagued the hospital. Buildings approached and in some cases surpassed obsolescence. By the 1980s, although some patients still lived on campus, most were transferred to clinics, nursing homes and foster homes. Small group therapy sessions represented a new system of outpatient care.

Buildings once intended to provide inpatient care were repurposed over the years as outpatient facilities. In some cases, medical research advances meant major changes in prognoses for patients. For example, the widespread use of penicillin for the treatment of syphilis meant a vast reduction in cases of neurosyphilis, the late stage of the disease marked by a deterioration of brain function. Through the 1930s, up to 10 percent of the patients at St. Elizabeths had syphilis. These numbers fell precipitously by midcentury, helping to reduce the numbers of people needing long-term residential care.

The patient population shrank, but the site remained a working hospital with a large staff. As a community clinic, the hospital divided its population

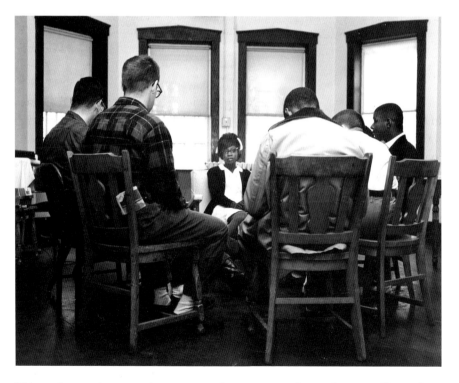

This small group therapy session represented a new system of outpatient care. *Photograph, circa 1970s, National Museum of Health and Medicine.*

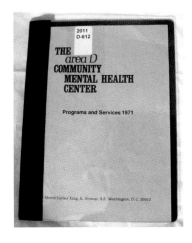

2011
D-612

THE
area D
COMMUNITY
MENTAL HEALTH
CENTER

Programs and Services 1971

Martin Luther King, Jr. Avenue, S.E. Washington, D.C. 20032

A new clinic with special programs for youth, alcohol and drug addiction and suicide prevention opened on the St. Elizabeths campus in the early 1970s. *From Programs and Services of the Area D Community Mental Health Center, brochure, 1971, U.S. National Library of Medicine. NBM staff photograph, 2018.*

into areas corresponding to the patients' original address. Emphasizing efficient, non-resident care, the clinic's outpatient programs aimed "to help people cope with mental or emotional problems as quickly as possible."[51] Perceived differences among Washington, D.C., neighborhoods informed the services provided in each area. A new clinic with special programs for youth, alcohol and drug addiction as well as suicide prevention opened on the St. Elizabeths campus specifically to treat the population of Area D in Southeast D.C.

St. Elizabeths went through a difficult transition during deinstitutionalization. The shrinking hospital was mired in bad publicity. In 1972, *Washington Post* reporter Karlyn Barker checked into St. Elizabeths as an undercover patient to get an unfiltered look at what went on inside its walls, in a Nelly Bly–like scheme. "I spent five days and five nights in a mental hospital," Barker wrote. "That's a genteel term for madhouse, but there was nothing genteel about being a sane person living among the insane." Barker, who described her stay as "excruciatingly depressing and boring," recounted the eerie voices that kept her up at night and the smells that pervaded the hospital's long hallways. She noted that the patients she lived with were "mostly old and mostly black." The multi-part series detailed day-to-day misery, noting at the beginning of her tale that "what I saw among these people was gruesome."[52] It was not the pretty picture of lawns and empathy that Dorothea Dix had envisioned.

A tense incident erupted in 1980 when Cuban refugees, at the hospital awaiting psychiatric evaluation, temporarily seized control of one of the buildings. Although the event ended peacefully for the rest of the hospital's population, the 1980s and 1990s brought other, more lasting problems, including loss of funding and accreditation and a generally sinking reputation around the city. By the time the last of the old buildings closed and some were demolished, few in town lamented the loss.

In 1987, the District of Columbia government under Mayor Marion Barry took over management of St. Elizabeths hospital. The Center Building had

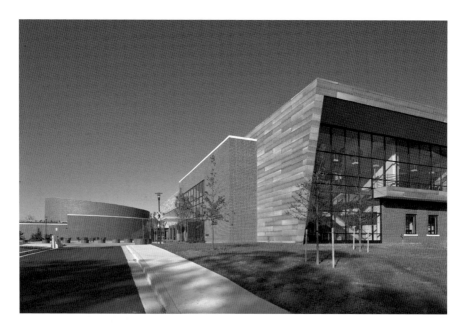

In 2010, Washington, D.C., consolidated all mental health care functions into a 293-bed hospital building, operated by the Department of Behavioral Health. *Photograph, 2010, architect EYP Architecture & Engineering, Turner Construction Company.*

been vacated beginning in the 1970s and was emptied of all personnel by 2003. While outpatients had continued to be seen for treatment in some of the smaller buildings, all patients were moved out of the historic buildings on the West Campus, after which time the midcentury structures on the East Campus were emptied of patients as well. In 2010, the city consolidated all mental health care functions into a new 293-bed hospital building, operated by the D.C. Department of Behavioral Health. The hospital offers both inpatient and outpatient treatment services, and it includes a learning apartment where patients train to leave the hospital and live on their own.

ST. ELIZABETHS EAST

When the Government Hospital for the Insane opened in 1855, and for many decades afterward, it operated on the rural fringe of the city. The site was surrounded mainly by farms, cemeteries and a military installation. Several Jewish congregations such as Adas Israel and Washington Hebrew purchased adjacent land for use as a cemetery, sited next to the hospital's cemetery on the East Campus. The Giesboro Cavalry Depot operated nearby, providing horses to the military during the Civil War. In 1911, Bolling Air Field, now Joint Base Anacostia–Bolling, was established on the western border of the campus, on the mud flats along the Potomac River.

Even when Southeast Washington burgeoned with residential neighborhoods such as Congress Heights in the early twentieth century, St. Elizabeths developed separately from its surrounding area. Most of the hospital was always inaccessible from local streets, surrounded by walls and fences. Local residents complained about escapees and patients with day passes wandering the streets, as well as about sights and odors coming from the farm. The hospital was simultaneously in the neighborhood and separate from it.

Meanwhile, the adjacent neighborhoods continued to change. Although the Civil War hindered city developers' early interest in a planned bedroom community on the east side of the Anacostia River for Navy Yard workers, the neighborhoods grew with the population of the capital city. Uniontown, a neighborhood now also known as the Anacostia Historic District, was platted in 1854. Barry Farm, north of the hospital, was funded by the Freedmen's Bureau beginning in 1867 and populated by both formerly enslaved and freeborn African Americans. By the 1920s and '30s, whites-only residential areas had developed at the end of the city streetcar line in Congress Heights, south of the hospital. All of these communities had ties to the hospital, with some families working at the site over several generations.

In the late 1960s, civil unrest rocked the nation's capital, as was true in cities throughout the country. And as in other major cities, Washington subsequently went through a period of white flight. Most white residents left Southeast seeking suburbanization and avoiding school and neighborhood integration. This major demographic change took place simultaneously with deinstitutionalization at the hospital, a major regional employer, meaning that the neighborhood experienced significant job loss as well. Since the 1970s, the neighborhoods around St. Elizabeths have been almost entirely African American. As one marker of such change, local residents celebrated in 1971 when Nichols Avenue, named after the hospital's first superintendent, was renamed Martin Luther King Jr. Avenue. The District Council called the new street name "a small but important step in focusing attention on the plight of Southeast Washington."[53]

In this period, throughout the city, citizens activated on many fronts to claim representational government. Demands for home rule led to an

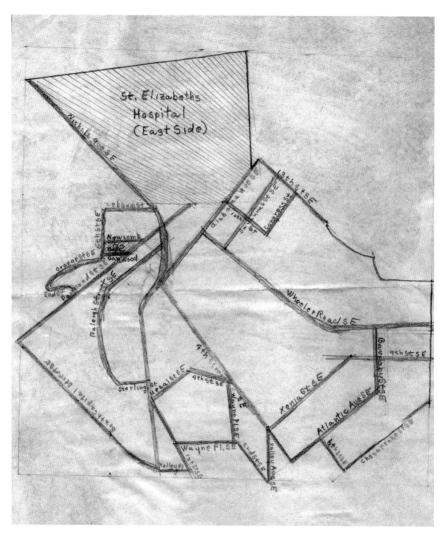

Statistician John Wymer noted that the neighborhood around St. Elizabeths was a "thinly settled area" dominated by the hospital to the north and "a white residential district" to the south. *Wymer map, 1948, John P. Wymer Photograph Collection, Historical Society of Washington, D.C.*

elected mayor and city council in 1974. To facilitate home rule, the new city council divided D.C. into eight wards, a system originating in the nineteenth century. The hospital campus sits at the intersection of Ward 7 and Ward 8, east of the Anacostia River.

For Washington, D.C., residents, the historic site on the East Campus, rebranded as St. Elizabeths East, presented abundant opportunities. In the 1970s and 1980s, as hospital functions retreated from deteriorating historic buildings, the city council and mayor's office explored different ways to reuse the campus. The city finally took control in 1987 following negotiation between Mayor Marion Barry and President Ronald Reagan. Redevelopment at this site, however, was slow to arrive. Reasons included disagreement on what redevelopment should look like, as well as municipal and private disinvestment in this low-income African American neighborhood across the river from the rest of the city. Efforts to redevelop the East Campus for mixed use intensified three decades later, after the federal government began to plan in earnest in 2002 for the future arrival of the Department of Homeland Security on the West Campus.

Washington, D.C.'s planned development at St. Elizabeths' East Campus has the potential to bring city investment to the area. However, with this new attention comes concern about gentrification and displacement, common concerns and realities for affordable housing advocates in other District neighborhoods. Near the corner of Malcolm X and Martin Luther King Jr. Avenues, SE, in Congress Heights, right across the street from the fenced-in hospital grounds, a mural illustrates Dr. King's inspirational quotation: "Only when it is dark enough, can you see the stars." The mural acknowledges the area's poverty and other problems and alludes to the hope that coming development will provide a bright new future for the region.

Several mayors have made plans to develop this vacant parcel of land and buildings, without much progress. Ideas included a hospital to replace D.C. General Hospital (formerly Gallinger, which had sent many patients to St. Elizabeths), which closed in 2001; a technology and innovation center; and a campus for the University of D.C. In 2012, children from Ward 8 participated in an art contest to imagine the new development on the East Campus. Entries included plans for a skate park, a retirement home, a Walmart, a daycare, a Martin Luther King Jr. Museum and plenty of roads in and out of the neighborhood. Meanwhile, the historic buildings have remained empty, enduring scavengers, waiting for rehabilitation and reuse.

Mayor Vincent Gray's 2014 plans for development at St. Elizabeths East called for a technology innovation hub for the city. As the first part of that plan, one of the first renovation projects transformed the 1955 St. Elizabeths Chapel, the realization of Chaplain Bruder's dream, into a modern technology center. The chapel's pews and stained-glass windows were replaced with whiteboards and desks for classroom use. The acronym RISE stands for "REL8 INOV8 STIMUL8 ELEV8" and symbolizes the connection between the site and the revitalization of the District's Ward 8. The Digital Inclusion program at the

RISE Center provides computer classes and support, with a focus on seniors, small businesses and job seekers.

Another newcomer to the East Campus is the Gateway Pavilion. The Gateway is a temporary location for festivals, farmers' markets, educational programing and arts events. At its ribbon-cutting, Deputy Mayor Victor Hoskins noted of the project that "this structure and its build-outs will provide the amenities the community needs and, frankly, deserves."[54]

Mayor Muriel Bowser stepped up the renovation plans during her term. Extensive infrastructure studies determined the best proposals for transportation and utilities on the historic campus. Planners had to start from scratch—there had never been a comprehensive boundary study or any topographical mapping done at the site. Neglect had led to corroded, out-of-date water systems. Years of rapid growth and haphazardly planned utilities revealed a tangle of sewers, electric and telephone lines, pipes and water mains across the entire campus, all of which needed to be addressed on both sides.

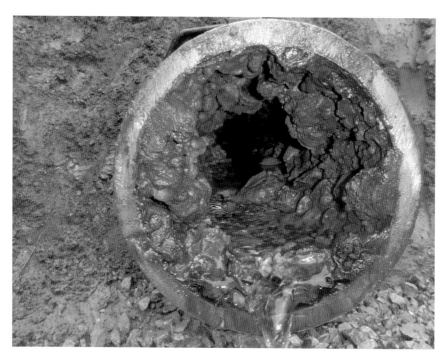

Extensive infrastructure studies revealed the poor state of utilities on campus. *From* St. Elizabeths East Existing Infrastructure Condition Report, *2012, prepared for the Office of the Deputy Mayor for Planning and Economic Development by CH2M Hill.*

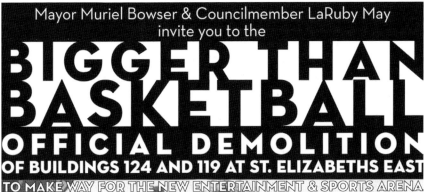

Mayor Muriel Bowser & Councilmember LaRuby May
invite you to the

BIGGER THAN BASKETBALL

OFFICIAL DEMOLITION
OF BUILDINGS 124 AND 119 AT ST. ELIZABETHS EAST
TO MAKE WAY FOR THE NEW ENTERTAINMENT & SPORTS ARENA

Address: 2700 Martin Luther King Jr. Ave SE
Date: Thursday, February 18th, 2016 | **Time:** 4:00PM
RSVP: biggerthanbasketball.eventbrite.com

Directions

From Alabama Ave SE:
  -Turn Right at 11th Place SE
  -Turn Left onto Dogwood Street
  -Make the first right toward Oak Street
  -Demolition event is 0.2 miles away

From MLK Ave SE:
  -Turn into campus on 2700 block of MLK Jr Ave
  -Turn right onto Dogwood Street
  -Make the first left toward Oak Street
  -Demolition event is 0.2 miles away

D.C. mayor Muriel Bowser invited the public to the demolition of two of St. Elizabeths East's mid-twentieth-century buildings. *Demolition announcement poster, 2016, Office of the Deputy Mayor for Planning and Economic Development.*

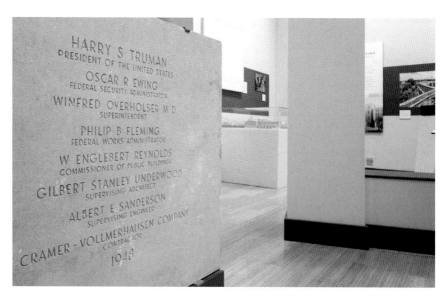

Many mid-twentieth-century structures were demolished to make way for a sports arena and other new development. *Cornerstone for Building 119, mid-twentieth century, Office of the Deputy Mayor for Planning and Economic Development. Photo by Yassine El Mansouri, 2017.*

In 2016, Mayor Bowser invited the public to the demolition of two mid-twentieth-century buildings. Haydon Hall, the geriatric patient building constructed in 1952, and the Rehabilitation Medicine Building, constructed in 1963, both came down in the name of future development. Neither structure was included in St. Elizabeths' 1991 National Historic Landmark nomination. Mayor Bowser's office advertised that the demolition event would be "Bigger than Basketball," to remind residents about the new events center set to replace the demolished structures. Opened in the fall of 2018, the 4,200-seat facility holds concerts, sports and cultural events year-round and is the home court for the Washington Mystics and the practice facility for the Washington Wizards.

Although St. Elizabeths Hospital still welcomes patients for mental health treatment, the rest of the campus is changing. Many structures were demolished to make way for the sports arena and other new development, while other historic buildings will be reused. Plans for St. Elizabeths East now include the transformation of the Continuous Treatment Buildings, originally built in the 1930s and 1940s, into apartments with surrounding green space and trails; 80 percent of units are reserved for affordable housing. The bucolic, restful landscape that Dorothea Dix so admired will be experienced by future generations, albeit under different circumstances than she originally intended.

THE WEST CAMPUS

The historic Kirkbride Center Building from 1855, as well as all other buildings on the historic West Campus, were vacated by patients and staff over several decades beginning in the 1970s. The buildings were protected only haphazardly, with broken water pipes leading to extensive interior deterioration. Many of the abandoned papers and artifacts were claimed by local museums and archives, including the Smithsonian Institution, the National Library of Medicine, the American Architectural Foundation, the Library of Congress, the National Park Service, the National Archives and Records Administration, the National Museum of Health and Medicine and Howard University. Yet some furniture, files and personal belongings remained in the vacant structures, untouched for decades. Although most items were long since rescued, excavations prior to recent construction work uncovered artifacts that reveal details of patient life from previous decades.

The buildings on the West Campus, transferred back and forth among federal and municipal government agencies, sat vacant for many years as proposals abounded for this prime real estate overlooking the confluence of the two rivers. One 1991 pitch for a new development called Rehoboth Village comprised a "planned, integrated, model community" in which

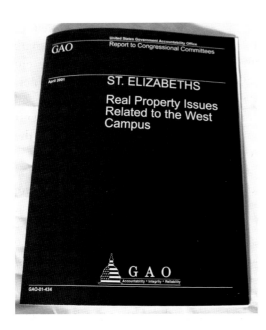

The West Campus was transferred to the U.S. General Services Administration (GSA) in 2004 after all patient care operations had been moved to the East Campus. *From* Real Property Issues Related to the West Campus: Report to Congressional Committees, *U.S. Government Accountability Office, 2001, National Library of Medicine. NBM staff photograph, 2018.*

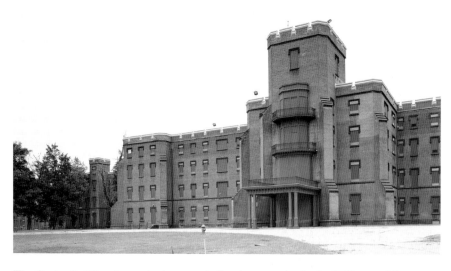

The Center Building, increasingly vacated of patients starting in the 1970s, was fully emptied of patients and staff in the 1990s. In many rooms, furniture, papers and personal belongings remained, untouched, for decades. *Photograph, circa 2000, © Carol Highsmith.*

"persons with mental or other handicaps" would live in a thriving mixed-use neighborhood alongside middle-income homeowners.[55] Although it owned the property briefly, the municipal government did not move forward with plans. Finally, in 2001, with all patient care operations moved to the East Campus, the West Campus was declared "in excess of need" for the U.S. Department of Health and Human Services and in 2004 was transferred to the U.S. General Services Administration (GSA), the agency that manages government properties, for use as a highly secure federal facility.

GSA surveyed the campus and prepared a master plan following vigorous debate and input from community residents and organizations, historic preservation and environmental advocates and federal and local government agencies. By this time, a new federal agency, the U.S. Department of Homeland Security (DHS), had been created and required a large parcel of land on which to consolidate its headquarters operations. GSA's 2009 master plan included the development of a high-security federal worksite on the West Campus.

DHS was founded in 2002 in part to improve interagency communication after the terrorist attacks of September 11, 2001. The agency's mission is to "prevent attacks and protect Americans on land, sea and air." DHS consolidated twenty-two preexisting government departments that had

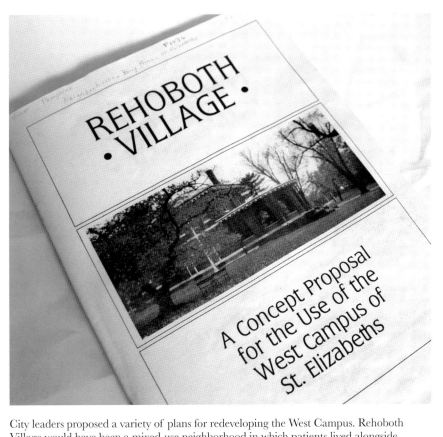

City leaders proposed a variety of plans for redeveloping the West Campus. Rehoboth Village would have been a mixed-use neighborhood in which patients lived alongside middle-income homeowners. *From* Rehoboth Village: A Concept Proposal for the Use of the West Campus of St. Elizabeths, *pamphlet, 1991, Historical Society of Washington, D.C. NBM staff photograph, 2018.*

been spread across the region. Looking to bring DHS headquarters and some of the component agencies together on one campus, GSA—not unlike Dorothea Dix in a previous century—studied the city looking for the best possible tract of land. Besides the river views and bucolic landscape, St. Elizabeths now also has access to both public transit and interstate highways for commuter transportation, as well as a campus that could accommodate perimeter security.

The first new structure to be completed on the West Campus was the headquarters of the U.S. Coast Guard, designed by Perkins + Will and completed in 2013. One of the largest construction projects in the region since the Pentagon, the LEED Gold-Certified building has one of the largest green roofs in the world and a constructed wetland.

Gatehouse 1 is a publicly visible building on the West Campus, having welcomed visitors for more than 150 years. Built in 1874, the structure is a mix of materials and patterns, a hallmark of the Queen Anne style. The rehabilitation of the gatehouse included reconstruction of a missing portico, based on an old photograph. The gatehouse now welcomes staff and visitors to the DHS campus.

Redevelopment of the West Campus for federal office space meant thousands of workers needing a cafeteria, and GSA responded by returning the 1885 Dining Hall to its original use. The LEED Silver-Certified structure reopened in 2013. Additional historic buildings are planned for adaptive use.

As the oldest and most significant structure on campus, the rehabilitated Center Building remains the focal point. Extensive archaeological, archival and architectural research has shaped the redevelopment process. Transforming a nineteenth-century building that was designed for patient wards and staff apartments into modern office space necessitated major

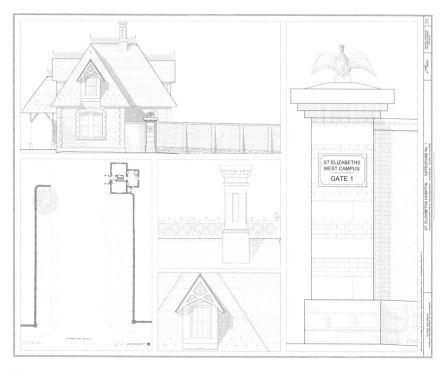

Prepared as part of GSA's documentation and rehabilitation of the historic West Campus, this 2017 measured drawing illustrates the gatehouse's placement at the main entrance. *Measured drawings, Historic American Buildings Survey (HABS), DC-349-AV, after 1933 National Park Service; Ita Ekanem, Scott Schwartz and Namrata Barbhaiya, Mills + Schnoering Architects.*

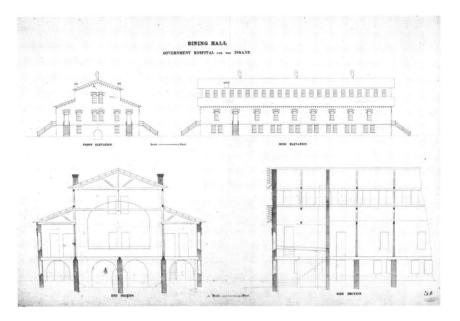

The dining hall could seat six hundred patients. *Drawing, 1885, Library of Congress, American Architectural Foundation Collection.*

design and structural intervention. Historical features such as door transoms, decorative trim and fireplace surrounds were preserved and reused in the most significant rooms and corridors. The building's exterior and core of the interior retain their original character. Significant interior spaces are embellished with stenciling, original grilles and trim salvaged from the building or replicated to echo their mid-nineteenth-century appearance. A newly constructed wing to the south of the Center Building complements the historic building.

The St. Elizabeths campus is a National Historic Landmark historic district, significant for its architecture, landscape and views, as well as the history of the hospital and its founders. The future of the historic district fueled several years of strong debate among interest groups and public agencies before the master plan was approved by the National Capital Planning Commission in 2009. The first phase of construction was funded that year by the American Recovery and Reinvestment Act.

Today, with the first phases of rehabilitation complete, GSA is continuing implementation of the master plan to build out the West Campus and preserve and rehabilitate as many of the site's character-defining buildings and features as possible. The defined historic landscape is protected as well.

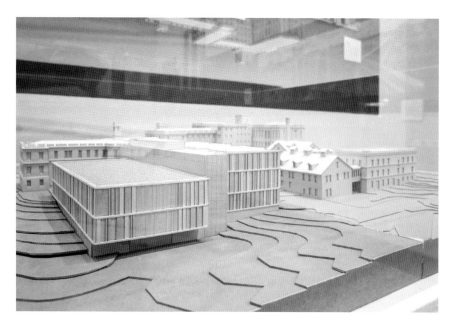

The West Addition, which is lightly attached to the Center Building, is an example of new construction on the historic campus. *West Wing addition model, proposed structure, 2016, Goody Clancy U.S. General Services Administration. Photo by Yassine El Mansouri, 2017.*

Additional information dating to early settlement of the land has come to light through archaeological investigation, promoting new interest in the site's early history.

As its buildings on both the East and West Campuses undergo extensive rehabilitation and reuse, St. Elizabeths enters a new chapter, with new types of land use and new opportunities for city residents and workers. City and federal leaders hope that this environment, once intended to cure the most vulnerable citizens, can now provide security, community and opportunity to future generations.

EPILOGUE

St. Elizabeths holds an important place in Washington, D.C., history. As the campus consolidated, archives, libraries, historical societies and museums across the city stepped in to preserve the past—each institution realizing the value of the historic material. In 2017, an exhibition exploring the history of St. Elizabeths opened at the National Building Museum in Washington, D.C. For the first time, "Architecture of an Asylum: St. Elizabeths, 1852–2017" brought together documents and artifacts from collections throughout the capital region to tell the story of the hospital. Over the course of the exhibition's ten-month run at the museum, more than fifty thousand visitors toured its galleries.

The multidisciplinary exhibition traced St. Elizabeths' evolution, reflecting shifting theories about how to care for the mentally ill, as well as the campus's later reconfiguration as a mixed-use urban development. An important collection of architectural drawings held by the Library of Congress anchored the exhibition, along with a series of architectural elements from the Center Building salvaged during rehabilitation by GSA. Drawings included Thomas U. Walter's plans for the institution's first structure, the 1855 Center Building, as well as plans for later residential cottages, farm structures and an auditorium. A spectacular 1904 model created to showcase the hospital at the St. Louis World's Fair served as a dramatic exhibition centerpiece.

Supplementing drawings and models included a wide variety of objects, from an electroshock machine to a patient-made cat sculpture, introducing

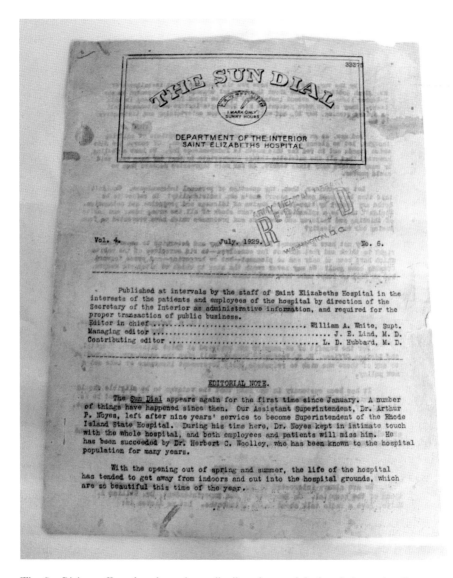

The *Sun Dial*, a staff-produced newsletter distributed around the hospital occasionally between 1917 and 1929, included pieces by employees and patients. *From the* Sun Dial, *pamphlet, 1929, U.S. National Library of Medicine. NBM staff photograph, 2018.*

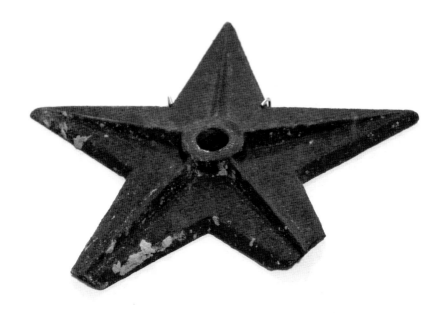

Building façade stars helped hold structures together by connecting iron bars between walls. *Building star, U.S. General Services Administration. NBM staff photograph, 2018.*

visitors to the people who lived and worked at the institution. Architectural fragments displayed from the recent renovations at the hospital complex included doors, ventilation grilles and paintings carefully cut out from the plaster walls before demolition.

In 2017, the exhibition at the National Building Museum presented a remarkable story about American healthcare, architectural history and promising adaptive use. Visitors were fascinated by the complex history of this hospital. This book honors and remembers Washington, D.C.'s first dedicated public mental health hospital and anticipates the contributions of this revitalized historic site to its neighborhood and to the city.

NOTES

Part I

1. National Alliance on Mental Illness, "Mental Health Conditions," https://www.nami.org/Learn-More/Mental-Health-Conditions.
2. Amariah Brigham, "The Moral Treatment of the Insane," *American Journal of Insanity* (March 1847).
3. British Library, "Illustration of Bedlam, by William Hogarth, 1735," https://www.bl.uk/collection-items/illustration-of-bedlam-by-william-hogarth-1735.
4. Shomer S. Zwelling, *Quest for a Cure: The Public Hospital in Williamsburg, 1773–1885* (Williamsburg, VA: Colonial Williamsburg Foundation, 1985), 5.
5. As quoted in Charles M. Synder, *The Lady and the President: The Letters of Dorothea Dix and Millard Fillmore* (Lexington: University Press of Kentucky, 1975), from a letter from Dorothea Dix to Anne Heath, undated, Dix mss., Harvard University.
6. As quoted in *The Dial* 11 (May 1880–April 1881).
7. Thomas S. Kirkbride, MD, *On the Construction, Organization, and General Arrangements of Hospitals for the Insane* (Philadelphia, PA, 1854).
8. John M. Galt, MD, *Journal of Insanity* (n.p.: April 1855).

Part II

9. March 3, 1855, CHAP. CXCIX, "An Act to Organize an Institution for the Insane of the Army and Navy, and of the District of Columbia, in the Said District," 33rd Congress, 2nd Session, C. 199, 1855.

10. Letter, Thomas Blagden to Dorothea Dix, November 13, 1852, as quoted in *Joint Select Committee to Investigate the Charities and Reformatory Institutions in the District of Columbia* (Washington, D.C.: Government Printing Office, 1898).

11. "Report of the Board of Visitors, Government Hospital for the Insane," in *Executive Documents of the House of Representatives for the Third Session of the Forty-Sixth Congress* (Washington, D.C.: Government Printing Office, 1881).

12. *Annual Report of the Department of the Interior, for the Fiscal Year Ending June 30, 1904.*

13. Copy of the appointment of Dr. Charles H. Nichols as superintendent of the Insane Asylum, Executive Documents printed by order of the Senate of the United States, 32nd Congress, 2nd Session, 1852–53.

14. "Report of the Secretary of the Interior," 36th Congress, 2nd Session, December 17, 1860.

15. "Report of the Secretary of the Interior, Communicating, in Compliance with a Resolution of the Senate, Information as to the Steps Taken to Establish a Lunatic Asylum in the District of Columbia," 32nd Congress, 2nd Session, December 30, 1852.

16. "Message from the President of the United States to the Two Houses of Congress," 36th Congress, 2nd Session, December 4, 1860.

17. Charles Nichols, Report to the Board of Directors, October 1, 1858, as quoted in Historic Preservation Review Board Application for Historic Landmark or Historic District Designation, 2009.

18. "Message from the President of the United States to the Two Houses of Congress," 35th Congress, 2nd Session, December 11, 1858.

19. Kirkbride, *On the Construction, Organization, and General Arrangements.*

20. Ibid.

21. "Report of the Government Hospital for the Insane," in "Message from the President of the United States to the Two Houses of Congress," 36th Congress, 1860.

22. Kirkbride, *On the Construction, Organization, and General Arrangements.*

23. "Message from the President of the United States to the Two Houses of Congress at the Commencement of the Second Session of the Thirty-Third Congress, Part I," 33rd Congress, 2nd Session, December 4, 1854.

Part III

24. "Report of the Board of Visitors of the Government Hospital for the Insane," 52nd Congress, 1st Session, October 1, 1891.

25. Ibid., 50th Congress, 1st Session, October 1, 1887

26. *Washington Post*, March 21, 1911.

27. *Report of the Committee to Consider the Organization and Needs of the Government Hospital for the Insane to the Secretary of the Interior* (Washington, D.C.: Government Printing Office, 1911).

28. *Report of the Committee to Consider the Organization and Needs of the Government Hospital for the Insane to the President of the United States* (Washington, D.C.: Government Printing Office, 1912).

29. "Government Hospital for the Insane, F.L. Olmsted, Jr., December 26, 1900," notes, Records of the Olmsted Associates, Series B, Job Files, job no. 2825, reel 135, frame 634.

Part IV

30. "Message from the President of the United States to the Two Houses of Congress at the Commencement of the Second Session of the Thirty-Third Congress, Part I," 33rd Congress, 2nd Session, December 4, 1854.

31. As quoted in Yanni, *Architecture of Madness*, 69.

32. *St. Elizabeths Hispanic Program: Culture-Specific Inpatient/Outpatient Care*, report, circa 1980, National Library of Medicine.

33. "Message from the President of the United States to the Two Houses of Congress," 34th Congress, 3rd Session, December 2, 1856.

34. "A True Statement of Affairs at St. Elizabeths Hospital for the Insane," in *Hearings Before the Special Committee Appointed by the Speaker Under a Resolution of the House of Representatives, Fifty-Ninth Congress, to Make a Full and Complete Investigation of the Management of the Government Hospital for the Insane* (Washington, D.C.: Government Printing Office, 1906).

35. From a letter from Superintendent Charles Nichols to Dorothea Dix, 1869, as quoted in Tomes, *Art of Asylum-Keeping*.

36. *By-Laws and Rules and Regulations of the Board of Visitors of the Government Hospital for the Insane* (Washington, D.C., 1900).

37. Administrative files, circa 1921–64, National Archives and Record Administration, Record Group 418, Entry 7, "Memoranda Incoming, 1953–1956," April 24, 1956, box 24.

38. Testimony of Dr. Harry H. Hummer, *Hearings Before the Special Committee Appointed by the Speaker Under a Resolution of the House of Representatives, Fifty-Ninth Congress, to Make a Full and Complete Investigation of the Management of the Government Hospital for the Insane* (Washington, D.C.: Government Printing Office, 1906).

39. "Report of the Board of Visitors of the Government Hospital for the Insane," 49th Congress, 2nd Session, October 1, 1886.

40. *Washington Post*, "Scores of Women Patients at St. Elizabeths Use Facilities Monthly," September 9, 1928, 18.

41. *Annual Reports of Subordinate Units, 1919–66*, National Archives and Record Administration, Record Group 418, Entry 20, "Chaplain," July 14, 1948, box 8.

42. Prentice Taylor Papers, Archives of American Art, Washington, D.C.

43. Nursing student handbook, circa 1950s, National Institutes of Health, NIH Stetten Museum.

44. *Annual Report to the Secretary of the Interior* (Washington, D.C.: Government Printing Office, 1905).

Part V

45. President John F. Kennedy, Special Message to the Congress on Mental Illness and Mental Retardation, February 5, 1963.

46. Ibid.

47. Trans-Allegheny Lunatic Asylum, http://www.trans-alleghenylunaticasylum.com.

48. Kirkbridge Hall, "History," https://www.kirkbridehall.com/history.

49. Henri E. Cauvin, "New Building Could Mark New Era for St. Elizabeths Hospital," *Washington Post*, April 19, 2010.

50. *U.S. Department of Health, Education, and Welfare, Secretary's Advisory Group on the Future of St. Elizabeths Hospital*, Final Report, 1964, U.S. National Library of Medicine.

51. *Programs and Services of the Area D Community Mental Health Center*, brochure, 1971, U.S. National Library of Medicine.

52. Karlyn Barker, "5 Days Inside St. Elizabeths: Anguish, Boredom, and Despair," *Washington Post*, July 16, 1972.

53. *Evening Star*, "Sign of the Times," January 15, 1971.

54. Washington D.C. Economic Partnership, "Mayor Gray Breaks Ground on Innovative St. Elizabeths Development Project in the Heart of Ward 8,"

May 29, 2013, https://wdcep.com/news/mayor-gray-breaks-ground-on-innovative-st-elizabeths-development-project-in-the-heart-of-ward-8.

55. *Rehoboth Village: A Concept Proposal for the Use of the West Campus of St. Elizabeths*, pamphlet, 1991, Historical Society of Washington, D.C.

BIBLIOGRAPHY

Books

Bly, Nellie. *Ten Days in a Mad-House*. N.p., 1887. http://digital.library.upenn. edu/women/bly/madhouse/madhouse.html.

Otto, Thomas. *St. Elizabeths: A History*. Washington, D.C.: General Services Administration, 2013. http://stelizabethsdevelopment.com/docs/full_ history_of_st_elizabeths.pdf.

Payne, Christopher. *Asylum: Inside the Closed World of State Mental Hospitals*. Cambridge, MA: MIT Press, 2009.

Tomes, Nancy. *The Art of Asylum-Keeping: Thomas Story Kirkbride and the Origins of Modern Psychiatry*. Philadelphia: University of Pennsylvania Press, 1994.

Yanni, Carla. *The Architecture of Madness: Insane Asylums in the United States*. Minneapolis: University of Minnesota Press, 2007.

Websites

Asylum Projects. http://www.asylumprojects.org/index.php?title=Main_ Page.

GSA/Department of Homeland Security at St. Elizabeths' West Campus. http://www.stelizabethsdevelopment.com/index.htm.

Kirkbride Buildings. http://www.kirkbridebuildings.com.

National Historic Register. Nomination form for St. Elizabeths. https://planning.dc.gov/sites/default/files/dc/sites/op/publication/attachments/Saint%20Elizabeths%20Hospital%20HD%20NHL%20nom.pdf.

St. Elizabeths East. http://stelizabethseast.com and http://www.stelizabethseast.com/wp-content/uploads/2014/03/8.3-Saint-Elizabeths-Hospital-East-Campus-Historic-Resource-Survey-July-2011-pt1-1.pdf.

Videos

Greystone Demolition. YouTube. https://www.youtube.com/watch?v=djzHvoqBRbo.

St. Elizabeths East. YouTube. https://www.youtube.com/watch?v=4tgMJcoAtcg.

Washington Post. Information about *Voices from Within*. https://www.washingtonpost.com/local/video-diaries-reveal-life-for-those-committed-to-st-elizabeths/2011/01/28/ABYjP5Q_story.html?utm_term=.0c0b09717a02.

ABOUT THE AUTHOR

Sarah A. Leavitt is a curator at the National Building Museum in Washington, D.C. Her latest exhibitions include "Community Policing in the Nation's Capital: The Pilot District Project, 1968–1973"; "House & Home"; and "Evicted," which explores the crisis of low-income renter eviction and encourages active engagement. Recent exhibitions have included "Cool and Collected: Recent Acquisitions" and "Architecture of an Asylum." Her first show at the Building Museum explored the history of the parking garage. She previously worked at the history office of the National Institutes of Health, where she curated exhibitions about medical advances such as the spectrophotofluorometer, and at the Heritage Center at the University of Colorado–Boulder, where her exhibitions covered subjects from student athletics to the space program. She was a founding staff member of the Women of the West Museum. She is most recently the editor of *Taliesin Diary: A Year with Frank Lloyd Wright* (Norton, 2013) and is the author of *From Catharine Beecher to Martha Stewart: A Cultural History of Domestic Advice* (UNC Press, 2002), as well as several articles on subjects ranging from the history of the pregnancy test to online motherhood communities to the television show *Veronica Mars*. She is also the author of the photo essay *Slater Mill* (Arcadia Press, 1997). She sits on the National Historic Landmarks Committee of the National Park Service. Leavitt graduated from Wesleyan University, where her undergraduate thesis focused on the incarceration of "wayward" girls, and holds a PhD in American Studies from Brown University. She lives in Silver Spring, Maryland.

Visit us at
www.historypress.com